# COMBAT CHRONIC PAIN

*Unleashing the Power of Cannabis, NLP, and Hypnosis for Lasting Relief*

## IRENE A YORK AKA GREEN IRENE

**First Printing Edition, 2023**

**ISBN:** 9798865492672

**Imprint:** Independently published

# *Dedication*

*To the Wellness Warriors,*

*Your strength, support, and unwavering belief in the power of healing inspire me daily. This book is dedicated to each of you who, like true warriors, face chronic pain with courage and resilience.*

*And To Bear,*

*You've been a constant companion through the darkest of days, offering a comforting presence and a shoulder to lean on. You've helped me heal, and for that, I'm forever grateful.*

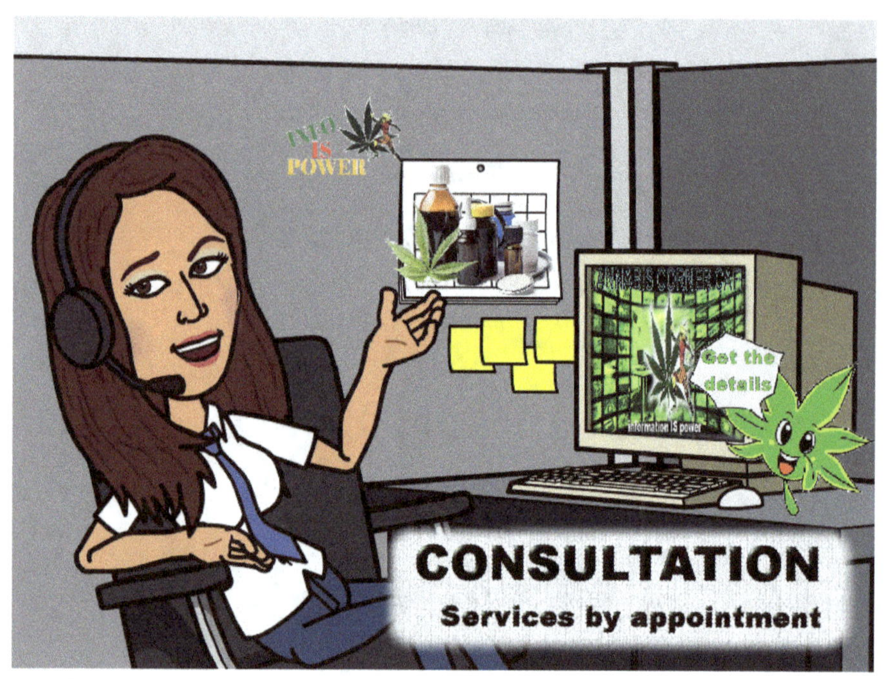
INFO
IS
POWER
CANNABIS CORNER CAFE
information IS power
Get the details
CONSULTATION
Services by appointment

# Table of Contents

## RECLAIMING HEALTH, WELLNESS & HAPPINESS



## EMPOWERMENT & INTEGRATION



## FINAL WORDS AND WISHES



## MORE INFORMATION & RESOURCES

# Author's Note

A Personal Journey of Healing and Empowerment

When I was first diagnosed with chronic pain (fibromyalgia and MS), my life took an unexpected turn down a winding road filled with frustration, despair, and countless medications that seemed to offer little relief. The debilitating pain and the accompanying emotional toll left me feeling helpless and trapped in a never-ending battle with my own body. Little did I know that my journey towards healing would lead me to write " the INFO-IS-POWER Series" to help others, like you – help you! This book is a reflection of my personal quest to not only overcome my chronic pain but also to empower others to take control of their pain management, pharma-free.

In the early days of my journey, I quickly realized that mainstream pharmaceutical approaches, though sometimes necessary, often came with a host of side effects that could be as troublesome as the pain itself. I longed for a more natural, holistic path to healing, one that would address the root causes of my pain rather than simply mask the symptoms. My journey led me to explore a variety of alternative therapies, and the three pillars that became the foundation of my practice, teachings, consultations, and books are cannabis, Neuro-Linguistic Programming (NLP), and hypnosis.

Cannabis, often misunderstood and stigmatized, has emerged as a powerful ally in the battle against chronic pain. The plant's natural compounds, known as cannabinoids, have been found to have potent analgesic properties, reducing pain without many of the side effects associated with traditional pain medications. However, my journey with cannabis was not without its own challenges. I navigated through the complex world of strains, dosages, and administration methods, all while adhering to the ever-evolving legal landscape of cannabis use. "Combat Chronic Pain" provides a comprehensive guide to understanding and utilizing cannabis as a pain management tool, ensuring that readers can access its benefits safely and effectively.

Neuro-Linguistic Programming (NLP), a field focused on the connection between language, thought, and behavior, played a crucial role in my journey. NLP techniques helped me reframe the way I perceived my pain and its impact on my life. It allowed me to break free from the cycle of negative thinking and self-limiting beliefs that had kept me stuck in a state of suffering in a wheelchair, or bed most of the time. In this book, I share specific NLP exercises and strategies that can help readers shift their mindset, regain control over their thoughts, and ultimately reduce their perception of pain. It's not about denying the existence of pain but about changing how we respond to it, making it a less dominant force in our lives.

Hypnosis, a practice often shrouded in mystery and misconceptions, was another transformative element of my healing journey. It's not about being manipulated by a mysterious figure swinging a pocket watch; it's about harnessing the power of the subconscious mind to influence our perception of pain. Through hypnosis, I learned to cultivate relaxation, reduce stress, and even manage pain more effectively. The book offers insights into what hypnosis is, how it works, and practical techniques and applications that you as the reader can use to engage with their own subconscious minds, enabling you to take charge of your pain experience.

But "Combat Chronic Pain" is not just a collection of techniques and knowledge. It's a deeply personal account of my journey, my struggles, my successes, and my setbacks. I share my own experiences, including moments of frustration and doubt, to let readers know that they are not alone in their pain. I understand the daily battles, the sleepless nights, and the overwhelming frustration that chronic pain can bring. My hope is that, through my story, readers will find solace and inspiration to embark on their path to healing.

The INFO-IS-POWER series, to which this book belongs, is all about providing readers with the knowledge and tools they need to become the first line of defense against *chronic any thing*. It's about empowerment, self-discovery, and reclaiming control over one's health. Rather than relying solely on pharmaceuticals, the series encourages readers to explore alternative, natural, and complementary approaches that can work in harmony with their bodies. "Combat Chronic Pain" embodies this philosophy by offering a roadmap for those seeking a more holistic approach to pain management.

Throughout the book, I emphasize the importance of working in partnership with professionals. While "Combat Chronic Pain" advocates for natural healing methods, it does not dismiss the value of traditional medicine. Instead, it encourages a more integrative approach where individuals can work alongside their doctors to develop a comprehensive pain management plan that considers both conventional and alternative therapies.

I want readers to know that "Combat Chronic Pain" isn't a one-size-fits-all solution. Each person's journey is unique, and what works for one may not work for another. However, the book provides a wealth of information and guidance to help readers tailor their own battle strategy, combining elements of cannabis, NLP, and hypnosis in a way that suits their individual needs and preferences.

In conclusion, "Combat Chronic Pain - A Battle Strategy Combining Cannabis, NLP, and Hypnosis" is not just a book; it's a lifeline for those who, like me, have experienced the daily struggle of chronic pain. It's a guide that offers both hope and practical solutions, empowering readers to become the first line of defense against their pain, pharma-free. My journey of healing led me to these powerful tools, and I believe they can lead others to a brighter, less painful future. Together, we can combat chronic pain, one page at a time.

# *Understanding the Enemy*

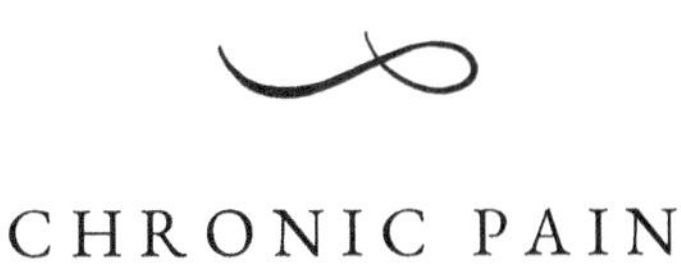

# CHRONIC PAIN

Chronic pain is an invisible burden that affects countless lives, including mine. It's a topic close to my heart, and I hope that by sharing my story, I can help shed light on what chronic pain is, its various forms, and how it drastically impacts a person's quality of life.

**Understanding Chronic Pain:**

Chronic pain, in its simplest form, is pain that persists for an extended period of time, typically lasting for more than 12 weeks. It differs from acute pain, which is your body's natural response to injury or illness, and typically resolves as the body heals. In contrast, chronic pain persists long after the initial injury or illness has healed. This ongoing pain can take various forms and can affect different parts of the body.

**Different Forms of Chronic Pain:**

Chronic pain doesn't discriminate, and it manifests in various forms. Some of the most common types include:

1. **Neuropathic Pain:** This type of pain arises from damage to the nervous system. It can feel like burning, tingling, or electric shocks and is commonly associated with conditions like diabetic neuropathy or sciatica.

2. **Musculoskeletal Pain:** This pain affects the muscles and joints. Conditions like fibromyalgia, osteoarthritis, and rheumatoid arthritis often cause musculoskeletal pain, making movement difficult and painful.

3. **Visceral Pain:** This is pain originating from the internal organs. Conditions like irritable bowel syndrome (IBS) and endometriosis can lead to chronic visceral pain, which is often challenging to diagnose and manage.

4. **Psychogenic Pain:** Sometimes, pain can persist due to emotional or psychological factors. While it doesn't have a clear physical cause, it is very real to those experiencing it. Conditions like somatic symptom disorder can lead to psychogenic pain.

5. **Mixed Pain:** Many individuals with chronic pain experience a combination of the above types, making diagnosis and treatment even more complex.

**The Distinction between Acute and Chronic Pain:**

One of the most critical distinctions between acute and chronic pain is the duration. Acute pain is your body's natural alarm system. It serves as a signal that something is wrong, and it's essential for our survival. For example, if you accidentally touch a hot stove, the sharp, intense pain you feel is acute pain. It's your body's way of saying, "Pull your hand away now!"

However, chronic pain is entirely different. It's like a broken alarm clock that won't stop ringing. Even after the initial injury or illness has healed, chronic pain persists. It becomes a constant companion, affecting not only your body but your mind and emotions as well.

Imagine having a headache that never goes away, a nagging, throbbing pain in your temples, day in and day out. Or consider living with relentless back pain, preventing you from bending, lifting, or even sleeping comfortably. These are just glimpses into the life of someone with chronic pain, and they barely scratch the surface of its effects.

**How Chronic Pain Affects the Quality of Life:**

Chronic pain has a profound impact on the quality of life of those who experience it. Let me share some insights into my journey and the daily challenges I face.

1. **Limitations on Physical Activities:** Chronic pain often restricts your ability to engage in physical activities you once enjoyed. For me, it meant giving up socializing, hiking, dancing, crafting, and so much more. The loss of these activities can lead to feelings of isolation and frustration.

2. **Emotional and Psychological Toll:** Living with chronic pain can take a significant toll on your emotional and mental well-being. It can lead to feelings of depression, anxiety, and even hopelessness. The constant discomfort, combined with the inability to do the things you love, can be emotionally draining.

3. **Social Isolation:** Chronic pain can lead to social withdrawal. You may find it challenging to make plans with friends or attend social gatherings, as unpredictable pain often makes it difficult to commit to activities. It certainly has played havoc with my social time and commitments to attend events etc.

4. **Sleep Disturbances:** Many chronic pain sufferers, myself included, experience sleep disturbances. The pain can keep you up

at night, and sleep deprivation exacerbates both the physical and emotional aspects of chronic pain.

5. **Work and Financial Impact:** Chronic pain can make it challenging to maintain regular employment. Some individuals may be forced to reduce their work hours or leave their jobs entirely, resulting in financial strain and instability.

6. **Medication Management:** Managing chronic pain often requires medications that can have side effects and potential risks. Finding the right treatment plan may involve a trial-and-error process, which can be frustrating and disheartening.

7. **Relationship Strain:** Chronic pain can put a strain on relationships. Loved ones may find it difficult to understand the constant struggle, leading to miscommunication and tension.

8. **Loss of Identity:** For many, chronic pain changes their sense of self. I used to define myself by my active lifestyle, but chronic pain forced me to reevaluate who I am and what I can do.

Despite all these challenges, those of us living with chronic pain are incredibly resilient. We adapt, we find support networks, and we push through each day with unwavering determination.

I want to emphasize that the experiences of people with chronic pain can vary greatly. What I've described here is just a glimpse into the complex and multifaceted nature of chronic pain. Each person's journey is unique, and the impact on their life may differ significantly.

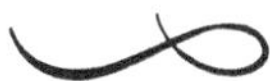

# THE IMPACT OF CHRONIC PAIN

Living with chronic pain has been a life-altering journey, and as I've walked this path, I've come to understand the profound physical and emotional toll it takes. Chronic pain is a relentless storm that sweeps through every aspect of your life, leaving behind its mark. In this personal narrative, I'll delve deeper into the impact of chronic pain, touching on the physical and emotional challenges I've faced and the pressing need for alternative solutions.

**The Physical Toll:**

One of the most palpable effects of chronic pain is the relentless physical toll it exacts. It's like carrying an invisible weight, a burden that never lifts.

Here's a glimpse of how it manifested in my life:

1. **Limitations on Physical Activities:** Chronic pain had, first and foremost, restricted my ability to engage in activities that once brought me joy. Simple tasks like walking, lifting, and even standing for extended periods of time became Herculean challenges. I used to love hiking in the great outdoors, yet, a gentle stroll left me in a state of agony.

2. **Daily Discomfort:** I would wake up every morning with pain as an unwelcome companion. It was there when I sat, or stood, even when I lied down. The pain didn't or wouldn't just stop at a dull throb; it often flared up, and often would become a searing, all-encompassing force that overshadowed everything else.

3. **Medication Dependency:** Managing chronic pain often involves a complex cocktail of medications, and I was prescribed a laundry list of Painkillers, anti-inflammatories, and muscle relaxants which became a part of my daily routine, bringing with them a slew of side effects and risks. Long-term medication use took its toll on my overall health, and I am still (10+ years later) recovering from some of the damage done from the pharmaceuticals I took.

4. **Sleep Disturbances:** One of the most insidious effects of chronic pain is its disruption of sleep. The pain often makes it difficult to fall asleep and stay asleep. The term "Night Owl" often could and still can be applied to me! (Admittedly, there is no quick fix.) Sleep deprivation, in turn, notably worsens the physical pain and deepens the emotional toll.

5. **Work and Financial Impact:** Chronic pain has affected my ability to maintain regular employment. I had to leave the traditional work force entirely causing a lot of financial hardships and instability. This financial instability and dependence on disability benefits added yet another layer of stress to the situation.

6. **The Daily Balancing Act:** Every day became a precarious balancing act, trying to manage the pain while fulfilling responsibilities. Sometimes still, I have to choose between meeting deadlines for a project, or managing my pain, and it's a choice I wish I didn't have to make.

**The Emotional Toll:**

Chronic pain isn't just about physical discomfort; it's a master of invading your emotional well-being. It reshapes your entire life's narrative.

Here are some of the emotional challenges I've encountered:

1. **Depression and Anxiety:** The constant pain is a breeding ground for depression and anxiety. It's difficult to remain upbeat and optimistic when pain is your constant companion. Simple tasks can become overwhelming, leading to feelings of despair and helplessness.

2. **Social Isolation:** I've often found myself retreating from social interactions. Chronic pain makes it challenging to make plans with friends, and the unpredictability of pain flares often means canceling at the last minute. It can lead to isolation and loneliness.

3. **Relationship Strain:** Chronic pain can put a strain on relationships. Loved ones may not fully grasp the daily struggle, leading to miscommunication and tension. Partners or Companions can sometimes experience an overwhelm and feel helpless which adds chaos and more strain. Sometimes, it feels like a barrier that separates you from those you care about.

4. **Identity Crisis:** For me, chronic pain has forced a re-evaluation of my sense of self. I used to define myself by my active lifestyle and independence, but chronic pain has required me to redefine

who I am. It's a difficult process of self-rediscovery – a journey along a long and winding road that can be challenging course.

5. **Lack of Understanding:** One of the most challenging aspects is the lack of understanding from others who haven't experienced chronic pain. It's difficult for them to comprehend the depth of suffering, which can lead to feelings of frustration and isolation, creating even more obstacles.

**The Need for Alternative Solutions:**

In the face of chronic pain's unrelenting assault on my life, I've explored various treatment options, from physical therapy to prescription medications. However, I've also come to realize that a multi-faceted approach is crucial. We need alternative solutions to manage chronic pain effectively.

1. **Complementary Therapies:** Alternative therapies like acupuncture, yoga, meditation, and chiropractic care have shown promise in managing chronic pain. While not a cure, they can provide some relief and improve overall well-being.

2. **Physical Rehabilitation:** Physical therapy and rehabilitation programs can help individuals regain some level of physical functionality. Learning how to move and exercise safely with chronic pain can be empowering.

3. **Pain Management Techniques:** Cognitive-behavioral therapy (CBT) and mindfulness techniques can be valuable in managing the emotional toll of chronic pain. As well as Neuro-Linguistic Programming techniques that teach coping strategies, relaxation, and ways to reframe negative thought patterns.

4. **Diet and Nutrition:** Some chronic pain conditions are exacerbated by inflammation. Exploring anti-inflammatory diets, can make a significant difference.

5. **Support Networks:** Support groups and therapy can provide emotional relief by connecting with others who understand the daily struggles of chronic pain. They offer a safe space for sharing experiences and seeking advice.

6. **Exploration of Alternative Medicine:** In many cases, alternative medicine, specific cannabinoids and terpenes lend themselves through Cannabis as a wonderful medicine that has proven potential in managing pain.

7. **Patient-Centered Care:** A holistic approach to pain management should prioritize the individual patient's needs and preferences. This means tailoring treatment plans to the specific circumstances and challenges of each person.

In conclusion, living with chronic pain is a journey through uncharted territory, one filled with physical and emotional challenges. The impact of chronic pain extends far beyond the physical realm, reshaping identity, and relationships. It's crucial to recognize the pressing need for alternative solutions and treatment approaches. Chronic pain is not a one-size-fits-all experience, and the solutions should be as diverse as the people it affects. As I continue to navigate this relentless storm, I remain focused on the research and innovation that will lead to more effective BATTLE STRATEGIES to COMBAT CHRONIC PAIN!

# *Cannabis – the healping herb*

# THE SCIENCE OF CANNABIS

As I sit down to write about the intriguing and evolving science of cannabis and its relationship with the endocannabinoid system (ECS) in the context of chronic pain, I can't help but reflect on how far we've come in understanding this remarkable plant and its potential to alleviate suffering. This journey through the world of cannabinoids, receptors, and chronic pain offers not only a glimpse into the cutting-edge science but also a testament to the profound impact that cannabis could have on countless lives.

Chronic pain, the uninvited guest that lingers long after its welcome has worn out, is a complex and debilitating condition that affects millions of people worldwide. For many, conventional pain management strategies have fallen short in providing sustainable relief. It's in this backdrop that the cannabis plant, particularly its active compounds called cannabinoids, has gained attention as an alternative for chronic pain sufferers. To fully grasp how cannabis works, it's essential to delve into the intricate world of the endocannabinoid system.

## The Endocannabinoid System: Our Body's Regulator

The endocannabinoid system is a fascinating network of receptors, endocannabinoids, and enzymes that plays a vital role in maintaining the body's internal balance, or homeostasis. It was discovered fairly recently in the late 80's early 90s, when scientists (Dr. Raphael Mechoulam and team) were trying to understand how THC, the psychoactive compound in cannabis, exerted its effects on the body. The revelation of this system opened doors to an entirely new field of research.

The ECS comprises three main components:

1. **Endocannabinoids**: These are naturally occurring compounds within our bodies that mimic the effects of cannabinoids found in the cannabis plant. Anandamide and 2-arachidonoylglycerol (2-AG) are two well-known endocannabinoids. They are produced on-demand in response to various physiological processes and function as signaling molecules.

2. **Cannabinoid Receptors**: There are two primary types of cannabinoid receptors: CB1 and CB2. CB1 receptors are mainly found in the brain and central nervous system, while CB2 receptors are more prevalent in the peripheral tissues, especially immune cells. These receptors act as gatekeepers, responding to endocannabinoids and external cannabinoids like THC and CBD.

3. **Enzymes**: Enzymes like fatty acid amide hydrolase (FAAH) and monoacylglycerol lipase (MAGL) break down endocannabinoids once their purpose has been served. This tight regulation ensures that the ECS remains responsive to changes in the body's needs.

## How the ECS Relates to Chronic Pain

In the context of chronic pain, the endocannabinoid system takes center stage. Pain, especially chronic pain, is often a result of inflammation or abnormal signaling in the nervous system. The ECS, with its intricate web of receptors and endocannabinoids, plays a crucial role in modulating these processes.

When the body experiences pain, endocannabinoids are synthesized on-demand and bind to cannabinoid receptors. CB1 receptors in the central nervous system can reduce pain perception, while CB2 receptors in peripheral tissues help to control inflammation and immune responses. This interaction helps restore the body's balance and alleviate pain.

But what happens when the body's endocannabinoids are not sufficient to address chronic pain? This is where cannabis comes into the picture.

## Cannabis and Chronic Pain: Unlocking the Potential

Cannabis contains over 100 different cannabinoids, with THC and CBD being the most well-known. THC is responsible for the psychoactive effects of cannabis, while CBD is non-psychoactive and has garnered considerable attention for its potential therapeutic properties.

THC, with its ability to bind to CB1 receptors in the central nervous system, can provide immediate pain relief by altering the perception of pain. This is particularly valuable for individuals suffering from conditions like neuropathic pain, where the nerves themselves are damaged and send pain signals uncontrollably. However, THC's psychoactive effects limit its use for many patients.

On the other hand, CBD has emerged as a promising candidate for managing chronic pain without the intoxicating side effects of THC. While CBD does not directly bind to CB1 or CB2 receptors, it influences the ECS in more subtle ways. It enhances the body's natural production of endocannabinoids, inhibits the breakdown of these compounds, or interacts with other receptors involved in pain perception.

Research on CBD's efficacy in pain management is still ongoing, but early studies and anecdotal evidence suggest its potential to reduce various types of pain, including neuropathic pain, inflammatory pain, and chronic pain associated with conditions like fibromyalgia and arthritis.

Moreover, the entourage effect, which suggests that different cannabinoids and terpenes in the cannabis plant work together synergistically, has piqued the interest of researchers. It implies that the therapeutic benefits of cannabis might be more significant when the whole plant is used, rather than isolated compounds.

## Challenges and Considerations

While the science of cannabis and the ECS holds great promise for chronic pain sufferers, it is not without challenges and considerations.

1. **Lack of Regulation**: The legal status of cannabis varies widely around the world, and even within regions where it is legal, the regulation of cannabis products can be lax. This makes it difficult for patients to access consistent treatments – to which I always tell patients – "Grow, grow, grow your own".

2. **Side Effects**: Cannabis, especially THC, can have side effects, including cognitive impairment, paranoia, and/or increased heart rate. It's essential to use the strain that is right for you, particularly for vulnerable populations – it is strongly advised that if you are new to cannabis consumption – seek the assistance of a reputable and knowledgeable Cannabis Consultant (I am available – www.greenirene.ca to book a call).

3. **Individual Variability**: Cannabis affects individuals differently due to factors like genetics, metabolism, and tolerance. Finding the

right strain and dosage can be a trial-and-error process though there is enough evidence to suggest strains that "typically help" patients in your condition.

4. **Stigma and Social Factors**: Sadly, there is still somewhat of an 'archaic attitude' and/or a stigma attached to cannabis use, even for medical purposes. Unfortunately, this can deter patients from exploring it as an option for pain management.

5. **Interactions with Medications**: Cannabis may interact with other medications a patient is taking, potentially leading to adverse effects. It's crucial for individuals to consult with healthcare and cannabis professionals before using cannabis as a pain management option.

**The Future of Cannabis in Pain Management**

As we move forward in the exploration of cannabis and the ECS for chronic pain, there is hope for a brighter future. With increasing legalization and the growing body of scientific research, patients have gained more access to safe and effective cannabis-based treatments as well as the right to grow their own medicine in most of North America.

In conclusion, the science of cannabis and the endocannabinoid system is shedding light on new avenues for chronic pain management. While challenges and uncertainties persist, the potential for improving the lives of those who have long suffered from chronic pain is a compelling reason to continue exploring this intriguing field. It is a testament to the resilience of science and human curiosity, as we unlock the secrets of this ancient plant and harness its potential to provide relief and healing in the modern world.

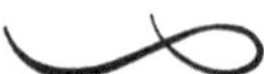

# CANNABINOIDS AND TERPENES

When it comes to alleviating pain, the cannabis plant has long been a subject of intrigue and controversy. Its complex chemistry, which includes a variety of cannabinoids and terpenes, offers an arsenal of relief for individuals suffering from chronic pain.

Among the most well-known components of the cannabis plant are THC (tetrahydrocannabinol) and CBD (cannabidiol), but there are many others, like CBG (cannabigerol) and CBC (cannabichromene), each with its own unique properties. In this exploration or section, we will delve into these components, understand how they work to alleviate pain, and identify predominant cannabis terpenes that have proven efficacy for chronic pain.

## Cannabinoids and Pain Relief

1. **THC (Tetrahydrocannabinol):** THC is perhaps the most famous cannabinoid, primarily responsible for the psychoactive effects of cannabis. It interacts with the endocannabinoid system (ECS) in the brain and body, binding to CB1 receptors, which are abundant in the central nervous system. This interaction can lead to the euphoric "high" associated with cannabis, but it also plays a significant role in pain management. THC can alter pain perception and reduce pain intensity by affecting the brain's processing of pain signals. It's particularly effective in managing neuropathic pain and pain associated with conditions like multiple sclerosis.

2. **CBD (Cannabidiol):** Unlike THC, CBD is non-psychoactive, making it a more attractive option for those who want pain relief without the "high." CBD does not directly bind to CB1 receptors but influences the ECS by enhancing the activity of endocannabinoids, such as anandamide. It can modulate inflammation, which is a common source of pain, and regulate pain perception by acting on TRPV1 receptors. CBD is known for its potential in reducing chronic pain, inflammation, and neuropathic pain.

3. **CBG (Cannabigerol):** CBG is one of the lesser-known cannabinoids but holds promise as an analgesic agent. It interacts with the ECS, mainly by binding to CB2 receptors, found in the immune system. CBG is believed to inhibit the uptake of GABA (gamma-aminobutyric acid), which can reduce muscle tension and pain. Furthermore, it can reduce inflammation and oxidative stress, contributing to its pain-relieving properties. Research on CBG is still in its early stages, but its potential for pain management is intriguing.

4. **CBC (Cannabichromene):** CBC is another non-psychoactive cannabinoid, often present in smaller amounts in cannabis strains. It doesn't directly interact with CB1 receptors but affects the ECS by interacting with TRPA1 and TRPV1 receptors, which play a role in pain sensation. CBC's ability to inhibit the uptake of anandamide can increase its concentration in the body, which, in turn, contributes to pain relief. It's particularly useful in managing chronic pain conditions, such as arthritis.

5. **THCV (Tetrahydrocannabivarin):** THCV is a lesser-known cannabinoid found in some strains of cannabis. While it is not typically considered a primary pain-reliever, it can indirectly aid in pain management by helping with weight management. Maintaining a healthy weight can reduce the strain on joints and, subsequently, alleviate pain in conditions like osteoarthritis. THCV can also influence the release of neurotransmitters, which may impact pain perception.

6. **CBDV (Cannabidivarin):** Like THCV, CBDV is not typically viewed as a direct pain reliever. However, it has shown promise in mitigating seizures in epilepsy, which can often be accompanied by neuropathic pain. Its anticonvulsant properties are noteworthy and may have applications in managing pain associated with neurological conditions.

## Terpenes and Pain Relief

In addition to cannabinoids, terpenes are aromatic compounds found in the cannabis plant, and they play a crucial role in the entourage effect, where the combined action of cannabinoids and terpenes produces a more significant therapeutic impact. Here are some predominant cannabis terpenes that have proven efficacy for chronic pain patients:

1. **Myrcene:** Myrcene is a terpene with a musky, earthy aroma and is commonly found in high concentrations in indica strains. It has strong analgesic and anti-inflammatory properties and can aid in muscle relaxation. Myrcene enhances the effects of cannabinoids like THC, making it a valuable component in pain management.

2. **Linalool:** Linalool is known for its floral and lavender-like scent. It possesses sedative and analgesic properties, making it effective in reducing pain and promoting relaxation. Linalool is often used to alleviate symptoms in conditions such as fibromyalgia.

3. **Caryophyllene:** Caryophyllene is a spicy terpene found in various cannabis strains. It has anti-inflammatory properties and selectively activates the CB2 receptor, which can help reduce pain and inflammation without the psychoactive effects often associated with THC.

4. **Pinene:** Pinene is a terpene with a piney aroma. It's known for its anti-inflammatory properties and can enhance cognitive function, which is particularly valuable for individuals dealing with pain-related cognitive impairment. Pinene can be found in both sativa and indica strains.

5. **Terpinolene:** Terpinolene is a terpene with a fresh, woody scent. It possesses sedative properties and can help reduce anxiety and pain. It's often found in strains that offer relaxation and pain relief without the intense psychoactive effects of THC.

**The Entourage Effect**

The entourage effect is a phenomenon where the various compounds in the cannabis plant, including cannabinoids and terpenes, work synergistically to produce a more potent therapeutic effect than any individual component could achieve alone. When it comes to pain management, this concept is crucial.

For example, a strain with a balanced combination of THC, CBD, and myrcene may offer better pain relief than a strain high in THC alone. The presence of CBD can mitigate the psychoactive effects of THC while myrcene enhances the analgesic properties. This illustrates the power of combining multiple cannabis compounds to address pain more effectively.

## Practical Considerations

When seeking pain relief through cannabis, several practical considerations should be kept in mind:

1. **Strain Selection:** Different cannabis strains contain varying combinations of cannabinoids and terpenes. Indica strains are often associated with relaxation and pain relief, while sativa strains may be more energizing. Hybrid strains can provide a balance.

2. **Dosing:** Finding the right dosage is essential. Start low and go slow to avoid potential side effects like anxiety or impairment. Consult with a professional experienced in medical cannabis – I am available and its easy to book a call through my website at www.greenirene.ca .

3. **Method of Consumption:** Cannabis can be consumed in various ways, including smoking, vaporization, edibles, and topicals. Each method has its onset time, duration of effects, and bioavailability, which can influence pain relief.

4. **Legal Considerations:** Cannabis laws vary by location. Ensure that you are compliant with local regulations and only purchase from reputable sources – or grow grow grow your own!

5. **Individual Variation:** How cannabis affects an individual can vary significantly. Factors such as genetics, tolerance, and overall health can impact the response to cannabis.

Bottom line is the cannabis plant offers a diverse range of components that have the potential to alleviate pain, from well-known cannabinoids like THC and CBD to lesser-known players like CBG and CBC. When combined with the right terpenes, the entourage effect can enhance the therapeutic benefits. However, it's essential to approach cannabis for pain management with caution, considering strain selection, dosing, and individual factors. Consulting with a professional experienced in medical cannabis can be invaluable in finding the most suitable approach for your unique needs. Pain management is a complex and personal journey, and cannabis is just one tool in the toolbox for those seeking relief.

# STRAIN SELECTIONS

For many people around the world, the pursuit of natural alternatives for pain relief has led them to explore the diverse world of cannabis strains. It helps to have some idea of what you might be looking for in terms of a strain name, strain profile, and/or strain effects. In this exploration, I share my top ten cannabis strains, which have gained popularity for their potential in alleviating pain.

1. **Cannatonic**:

    - **Cannabinoids**: Cannatonic is renowned for its high CBD (cannabidiol) content, often surpassing 12%, with very low THC levels (usually below 6%).

    - **Terpenes**: Myrcene, Pinene, and Caryophyllene are common terpenes found in Cannatonic, contributing to its mild, earthy aroma.

- **Effects**: With its high CBD and low THC ratio, Cannatonic is considered a "gentle giant." It provides pain relief without the intense psychoactive effects typically associated with cannabis.

- **Availability**: Cannatonic can be found in most medical and some recreational dispensaries where cannabis is legal.

2. **Remedy**:

- **Cannabinoids**: Remedy is another high-CBD strain, with CBD levels often exceeding 15%, while THC is minimal, generally less than 1%.

- **Terpenes**: Terpinolene, Myrcene, and Caryophyllene contribute to Remedy's unique aromatic profile, which combines hints of citrus and earthiness.

- **Effects**: Like Cannatonic, Remedy is favored for its ability to provide pain relief without the psychoactive "high." It's often chosen by those who seek relief from chronic pain and inflammation.

- **Availability**: Remedy is available in various legal cannabis markets, particularly in regions with robust medical cannabis programs.

3. **ACDC**:

- **Cannabinoids**: ACDC is another CBD-dominant strain, typically boasting CBD levels of 20% or higher and low THC, usually below 1%.

- **Terpenes**: Myrcene, Pinene, and Caryophyllene are common terpenes in ACDC, contributing to its herbal and earthy scent.

- **Effects**: ACDC is known for its relaxing effects and powerful pain-relieving properties. It's often sought after for various chronic pain conditions.

- **Availability**: ACDC can be found in both medical and recreational cannabis markets where CBD-rich strains are appreciated.

4. **AK-47**:

- **Cannabinoids**: AK-47 is a hybrid strain with moderate levels of both THC and CBD, with THC levels typically ranging from 13% to 20%.

- **Terpenes**: It features a complex terpene profile with hints of citrus, earthiness, and skunkiness.

- **Effects**: Despite its name, AK-47 is known for its calming and pain-relieving effects. Its balanced THC-to-CBD ratio makes it a favorite among those seeking relief from various types of pain.

- **Availability**: AK-47 is available in many cannabis markets, both for medical and recreational use.

5. **Blackberry Kush**:

- **Cannabinoids**: Blackberry Kush is an indica-dominant strain with moderate THC levels, often ranging from 16% to 20%, and minimal CBD content.

- **Terpenes**: It features terpenes like Myrcene, Caryophyllene, and Limonene, giving it a sweet, berry-like aroma.

- **Effects**: Blackberry Kush provides deep relaxation and is often used for pain management, especially for conditions involving muscle tension and insomnia.

- **Availability**: It's commonly available in areas with legal cannabis markets.

6. **Granddaddy Purple**:

- **Cannabinoids**: Granddaddy Purple is another indica-dominant strain with THC levels typically ranging from 17% to 23%.

- **Terpenes**: It's rich in Myrcene, Caryophyllene, and Pinene, contributing to its sweet and fruity aroma.

- **Effects**: Granddaddy Purple is prized for its relaxing and sedative effects, making it suitable for managing various types of pain and aiding sleep.

- **Availability**: This strain is widely available in the recreational and medical cannabis markets.

7. **White Widow**:

- **Cannabinoids**: White Widow is a balanced hybrid with moderate THC levels, ranging from 18% to 25%, and minimal CBD content.

- **Terpenes**: It contains terpenes such as Myrcene, Caryophyllene, and Limonene, giving it a pungent, earthy scent.

- **Effects**: White Widow is known for its euphoric and pain-relieving effects. It's a versatile strain that can help alleviate various forms of pain while maintaining mental clarity.

- **Availability**: White Widow is often found in both medical and recreational cannabis markets.

8. **Purple Arrow**:

- **Cannabinoids**: Purple Arrow is an indica-dominant strain with THC levels often exceeding 20%, and negligible CBD content.

- **Terpenes**: Terpenes like Myrcene, Caryophyllene, and Linalool contribute to its sweet and floral aroma.

- **Effects**: Purple Arrow is celebrated for its calming effects, making it effective in managing pain and stress, especially before bedtime.

- **Availability**: It can be found in regions with legal cannabis markets that appreciate indica strains.

9. **Blueberry Kush**:

- **Cannabinoids**: Blueberry Kush is an indica-dominant strain with THC levels typically ranging from 16% to 24%, and minimal CBD content.

- **Terpenes**: It features terpenes like Myrcene, Caryophyllene, and Pinene, giving it a sweet, fruity scent.

- **Effects**: Blueberry Kush is known for its relaxing and pain-relieving properties, making it a favorite for those suffering from chronic pain and stress.

- **Availability**: It's widely available in both medical and recreational cannabis markets.

10. **Black Domina**:

    - **Cannabinoids**: Black Domina is an indica-dominant strain with high THC levels, often surpassing 20%, and minimal CBD content.

    - **Terpenes**: It contains terpenes such as Myrcene, Caryophyllene, and Pinene, contributing to its earthy and spicy aroma.

    - **Effects**: Black Domina is prized for its powerful pain-relieving and sedative effects, making it a go-to choice for those dealing with severe pain and insomnia.

    - **Availability**: It can be found in regions with legal cannabis markets, often as a specialized strain due to its potency.

When it comes to alleviating pain, choosing the right cannabis strain involves considering the balance of cannabinoids and terpenes. High-CBD strains like Cannatonic, Remedy, and ACDC are preferred for those who want pain relief without the psychoactive effects of THC. However, strains like AK-47, Blackberry Kush, and Granddaddy Purple, which have moderate to high THC content, are also effective for pain management.

Terpenes play a crucial role in the aroma and overall effects of each strain. Myrcene, commonly found in many of these strains, contributes to their calming and sedative properties. Caryophyllene, which is also prevalent, has anti-inflammatory and pain-relieving qualities. Other terpenes, like Pinene, Limonene, and Linalool, add unique aromatic profiles and therapeutic benefits to these strains.

Availability of these strains can vary depending on your location and the legal status of cannabis. In regions with legalized medical and recreational cannabis, you're more likely to find a wider selection of strains. In regions where only medical use is allowed, you might need a prescription or medical card to access certain or specific strains.

Remember that the effectiveness of a particular strain for pain relief can vary from person to person. Individual responses are influenced by factors like the type and intensity of pain, personal tolerance, and overall health. It's crucial to consult with a professional to find the strain that best suits your needs and preferences. Keeping a journal or log of the strains you try can go a long way in helping you to help you!

On the next page you'll find an excellent example and template of a journal or log entry. Note, that a simple notebook from the dollar store is enough to help you keep track. However, I do have battle strategy Journals available for purchase on Amazon @ https://amzn.to/3sd7QNM

That said, in the world of cannabis - strains offers a diverse array of options for pain relief. Whether you prefer a high-CBD, low-THC strain like Cannatonic or a more balanced option like White Widow, there's likely a strain that can provide the relief you seek. As the cannabis industry continues to evolve, more strains tailored for specific therapeutic purposes are likely to emerge, providing even more choices for those looking to manage their pain naturally and effectively.

<table>
<tr>
<td>Example of Entries I've made in mine!</td>
<td>

**Journal Entry - Date: 6/23/2021**

**Before Consumption:**

</td>
</tr>
</table>

- Physical Condition: Feeling stressed and anxious due to a long workday.

- Method of Consumption: Vaporization using the Volcano vaporizer.

- Strain: Blue Dream

- Cannabinoids: THC 18%, CBD 2%

- Terpenes: Myrcene, pinene, caryophyllene

- Purchased from: Local Dispensary - "GreenLeaf Haven"

**During Consumption:**

- I took a few hits from the vaporizer and felt the soothing effects almost immediately. The taste was earthy and slightly sweet, with a hint of pine.

**After Consumption:**

- Physical Condition: About 15 minutes later, I noticed a significant reduction in stress and anxiety. My body felt relaxed, and my mood improved. There's a gentle euphoria without feeling overly sedated, making it a good option for evening use. My creativity seems to be enhanced, which is perfect for doing my hobbies.

- Strain Experience: I really enjoy this strain. It provides a nice balance between relaxation and focus. The mild CBD content seems to take the edge off the THC, preventing any unwanted anxiety. The terpenes give it a pleasant aroma and flavor, and I find it very enjoyable.

- Overall, it's a great strain for unwinding after a long day without feeling too spacey or tired.

> Example of Entries I've made in mine!

**Journal Entry - Date: 10/25/2022**

**Before Consumption:**

- Physical Condition: Dealing with a persistent headache and some muscle tension.

- Method of Consumption: Sublingual tincture - "ACME CBD Drops" from a local dispensary.

- Strain: CBD-dominant strain

- Cannabinoids: CBD 12%, THC 1%

- Terpenes: None specified

**During Consumption:**

- I measured out the recommended dose of the CBD tincture and held it under my tongue for a minute before swallowing. The taste was quite mild, with a hint of earthiness.

**After Consumption:**

- Physical Condition: About 30 minutes after taking the tincture, my headache began to ease, and the muscle tension in my neck and shoulders slowly diminished. There's no "high" associated with this strain due to the minimal THC content, but it provides great relief for my physical discomfort.

- Strain Experience: While I wouldn't consider this a recreational strain, it's excellent for managing pain and tension without any intoxicating effects. I appreciate its mild flavor and consistent results. It's become one of my go-to options for dealing with physical discomfort.

> Example of Entries I've made in mine!

**Journal Entry - Date: 2/27/2023**

**Before Consumption:**

- Physical Condition: Struggling with insomnia and high stress levels.

- Method of Consumption: Edibles - "Dreamy Delights" brand gummies, containing an indica strain.

- Strain: Purple Kush

- Cannabinoids: THC 20%, CBD 1%

- Terpenes: Linalool, myrcene, caryophyllene

- Purchased from: Local Dispensary - "GreenLeaf Haven"

**During Consumption:**

- I ate two gummies, each containing 25mg of THC. They tasted like berries and had a pleasant texture.

**After Consumption:**

- Physical Condition: It took about an hour, but eventually, I felt deeply relaxed and drowsy. My stress melted away, and I drifted off to sleep easily. The effects were long-lasting, and I woke up feeling refreshed.

- Strain Experience: Purple Kush is a fantastic choice for managing stress and insomnia. The gummies made consumption easy and discreet. I highly recommend this strain for anyone looking to unwind and get a good night's sleep.

Note: Please consult with a healthcare professional before using medical cannabis and follow local laws and regulations regarding its use. The strains and products mentioned in these examples are genuinely personal entries – remember cannabis affects everyone differently. I have provided these examples for illustrative purposes only.

The following is a template that you can imitate, or you can purchase the BATTLE STRATEGY 31 DAY JOURNAL (Single or in a pack of 3) from Amazon @ https://amzn.to/3sd7QNM

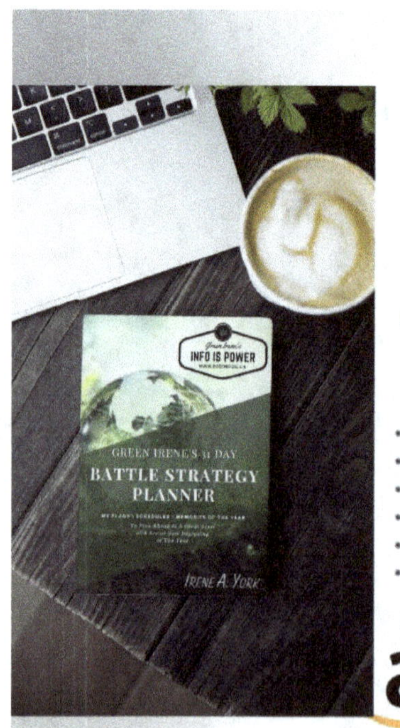

**Medical Cannabis Consumption Journal Template**

**Date:** [Date] **Patient Name:** [Your Name] **Medical Cannabis Consultant:** [If applicable]

**Entry #1:**

**Date:** [Date] **Time:** [Time] **Strain Name:** [Strain Name] **Method of Consumption:** [Method, e.g., Vaping, Edibles] **Cannabinoids:** [Cannabinoid content, e.g., THC: 20%, CBD: 1%] **Terpenes:** [Terpene profile, if known] **Dose:** [Amount consumed, e.g., 0.2 grams]

**Before Consumption:**

- **Physical Condition:** Describe any symptoms or conditions you're experiencing.

- **Mood:** Your emotional state.

**Effects or Relief:**

- **Immediate Effects:** Describe any immediate effects you feel after consuming.

- **Long-term Effects:** How do you expect this to affect your condition throughout the day?

**Strain Opinion:** [Like/Dislike]

**Purchase Location/Brand:** [Where you purchased it, or the name of the licensed producer (LP) brand]

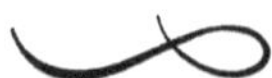

# DOSING AND TITRATION

In recent years, the landscape of cannabis consumption has transformed dramatically. As an advocate for the responsible use of this plant, I have seen firsthand the growing interest in cannabis for both medicinal and recreational purposes. However, with this increased interest comes a need for a deeper understanding of the key elements of a successful cannabis experience: strains, titration, and dosing.

## Cannabis Strains: A World of Diversity

One of the fundamental aspects of cannabis is the incredible diversity of strains available. Each strain possesses a unique combination of compounds, resulting in distinct effects on the user. The two primary species of cannabis, Cannabis sativa and Cannabis indica, as well as hybrid strains, provide an extensive spectrum of experiences.

1. **Sativa Strains**: Sativa strains are known for their energizing and uplifting effects. Sativas are ideal for daytime use, offering increased focus, creativity, and a boost in mood. Many users turn to sativa strains for activities that require mental clarity and alertness.

2. **Indica Strains**: Indica strains, on the other hand, are renowned for their relaxing and sedative qualities. Indica's are often chosen for nighttime use, helping with pain relief, anxiety reduction, and sleep.

3. **Hybrid Strains**: Hybrid strains combine characteristics of both sativa and indica varieties. The effects of hybrids can vary widely depending on the specific genetics of the strain. Some hybrids are balanced in their sativa and indica properties, making them versatile choices for a range of situations.

## Selecting the Right Strain

Choosing the right strain is a crucial step in responsible cannabis consumption. The choice should align with your individual needs and preferences. Here are some guidelines to help you select the most suitable strain:

1. **Consider Your Goals**: Start by identifying your goals for cannabis use. Are you seeking relaxation, pain relief, or enhanced creativity? Your goals will guide your strain selection.

2. **Understand Your Tolerance**: If you're a novice user, strains with lower THC content are recommended to avoid overwhelming psychoactive effects. Conversely, experienced users might opt for high-THC strains for specific purposes.

3. **Consult with a Budtender**: In regions with legalized cannabis dispensaries, budtenders can provide valuable guidance. They can

recommend strains based on your desired effects and personal history with cannabis.

4.  **Experiment and Keep a Journal**: Finding the right strain may require some experimentation. Keeping a journal like the examples above to record your experiences with different strains, dosages, and their effects. Will go a long way in helping you refine your choices over time.

## Titration: The Art of Finding Your Ideal Dose

Titration is the process of finding your ideal cannabis dosage to achieve the desired effects while minimizing potential negative outcomes. It's a personal journey, as tolerance, metabolism, and individual responses to cannabis can vary greatly. Here's how to approach titration:

1.  **Start Low and Go Slow**: Begin with a low dose, especially if you're new to cannabis or trying a new strain. Low doses minimize the risk of overwhelming psychoactive effects. You can always consume more if needed.

2.  **Wait and Observe**: After taking a small dose, wait at least 30 minutes to assess the effects. Cannabis affects individuals differently, and it might take time for the full impact to be felt.

3.  **Incrementally Adjust**: If the initial dose isn't achieving your desired effects, consider increasing it slightly in your subsequent session. Continue this process until you find your ideal dose.

4.  **Mind the Method**: The method of consumption also plays a role in titration. Smoking or vaporizing typically result in quicker effects, while edibles have a delayed onset. Be mindful of this when titrating.

5. **Avoid Bingeing**: It's crucial to avoid overconsumption. Bingeing on cannabis can lead to discomfort and a negative experience. Titration helps prevent this.

## Dosing Guidelines

Once you've found your ideal dose, it's important to understand dosing guidelines to maintain a safe and enjoyable experience. These guidelines can vary depending on your tolerance, the strain, and the method of consumption.

1. **Microdosing**: Microdosing involves consuming very small amounts of cannabis, typically around 2.5-5 milligrams of THC. This approach is ideal for enhancing creativity, focus, or managing chronic pain symptoms without significant psychoactive effects.

2. **Low Doses**: A low dose for most users ranges from 5-10 milligrams of THC. This dose is suitable for novice users and those seeking mild relaxation or pain relief without intense psychoactivity.

3. **Moderate Doses**: Moderate doses, typically between 10-30 milligrams of THC, offer a balance of therapeutic benefits and psychoactivity. They're suitable for users with some tolerance and specific needs.

4. **High Doses**: High doses, exceeding 30 milligrams of THC, should be approached with caution. They are generally reserved for experienced users with a high tolerance, particularly when using cannabis for severe pain or advanced medical conditions.

5. **CBD-THC Ratios**: When using strains with a balanced CBD-THC ratio, the presence of CBD can mitigate the psychoactive effects of THC. This is especially relevant for medical users seeking symptom relief without a pronounced high.

In the realm of cannabis consumption, strains, titration, and dosing are integral components of a successful and responsible experience. Selecting the right strain tailored to your goals and preferences is the first step. From there, titration helps you find your ideal dose, ensuring that you receive the desired effects without overindulging. Understanding dosing guidelines is the final piece of the puzzle, allowing you to maintain a safe and enjoyable relationship with cannabis.

The importance of approaching cannabis use with knowledge, respect, and responsibility cannot be overstated. It's through this approach that individuals can harness the full potential of this remarkable plant while minimizing potential pitfalls. By following these guidelines and staying informed, individuals can embark on a journey of self-discovery and wellness through cannabis, making the most of the diverse array of strains available to them.

# *Neuro-Linguistic Programming (N.L.P.)*

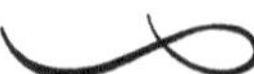

# THE WEAPON TO MASTER YOUR MIND

As I sit down to write this, I'm reminded of the countless moments I've spent in agony, the pain so relentless that it consumed my every thought and action. Chronic pain had become my unwanted companion, dictating my life, and leaving me feeling utterly powerless. However, my journey through the labyrinth of pain led me to a remarkable discovery - Neuro-Linguistic Programming (NLP).

This introduction to NLP aims to provide you with a profound understanding of what NLP is, its guiding principles, and its incredible relevance in managing chronic pain. NLP is not just a set of techniques; it's a philosophy, a science, and an art that can change the way you perceive and experience pain, ultimately enabling you to regain control over your life.

**Unveiling Neuro-Linguistic Programming (NLP)**

Neuro-Linguistic Programming, often referred to as NLP, is a versatile and transformative approach to understanding and improving human communication, behavior, and thought patterns. It was developed in the 1970s by John Grinder and Richard Bandler, drawing from the work of psychologists and linguists like Fritz Perls, Virginia Satir, and Milton H. Erickson. The core idea behind NLP is that by studying the thought processes and behaviors of highly successful individuals, we can model their strategies for success and apply them to our own lives.

But what does this mean for managing chronic pain?

Imagine this: Pain is not just a physical sensation; it's a complex interplay of sensory experiences, emotions, and thoughts. NLP recognizes that our perception of pain is not a fixed reality but a dynamic construct influenced by our neurology (neuro), language (linguistic), and the patterns we've developed over time (programming). With NLP, we can gain insight into how we create our pain experience and learn to reprogram our responses to it.

**The Principles of NLP**

1. **The Map is Not the Territory**: NLP asserts that each person's perception of the world is unique, and they construct their own reality. Our individual experiences are like maps, and these maps may not always accurately represent the objective reality, which is the territory. When dealing with chronic pain, this principle reminds us that our experience of pain is influenced by our unique perceptions, beliefs, and past experiences.

2. **Mind and Body Are Connected**: NLP recognizes the profound connection between our mental and physical states. Pain, especially chronic pain, is not solely a physical issue; it involves emotions, thoughts, and beliefs. By addressing the mind-body

connection, NLP techniques can help alleviate both the emotional and physical aspects of pain.

3. **Communication is Key**: NLP places a strong emphasis on effective communication. This includes the communication we have with ourselves (internal dialogue) and with others. When it comes to pain management, improving self-talk and communication can significantly reduce suffering and enhance resilience.

4. **Modeling Excellence**: One of the fundamental principles of NLP is modeling. This involves studying and replicating the thought and behavioral patterns of those who have achieved success in a particular area. In the context of chronic pain, modeling can help us learn from individuals who have effectively managed their pain and apply their strategies to our own lives.

## Relevance of NLP in Managing Chronic Pain

Now, you may be wondering, "How can NLP help me with my chronic pain?" Let's delve into the ways NLP techniques and principles can be applied to alleviate suffering and regain control over your life.

## 1. Reframing Your Pain Narrative

One of the most powerful tools in the NLP toolkit is reframing. NLP encourages you to view your pain from different perspectives, altering the meaning and emotional charge attached to it. By changing how you frame your pain, you can reduce the intensity of your suffering. For instance, instead of seeing your pain as an enemy that must be fought, you can reframe it as a teacher that offers lessons in resilience and strength.

## 2. Mind-Body Connection and Visualization

NLP teaches us to harness the power of our mind-body connection. Through visualization and guided imagery techniques, you can use the power of your imagination to reduce pain. By creating positive, pain-free mental images, you signal your body to respond accordingly. This is not about wishful thinking; it's about rewiring your neurological responses to pain.

## 3. Anchoring for Pain Management

Anchoring is an NLP technique that associates a specific stimulus with a desired emotional state. It can be used to create a pain-free or relaxed state in response to a particular trigger. For instance, you can create an anchor by touching a specific part of your body when you are in a state of minimal pain or relaxation. With practice, you can trigger this anchor to reduce pain when it's most needed.

## 4. Language and Self-Talk Transformation

The way we talk to ourselves can either exacerbate or alleviate our pain. NLP helps you become aware of your internal dialogue and, if necessary, change the language you use to describe your pain. Instead of saying, "I'm in excruciating pain," you can shift to statements like, "I'm experiencing discomfort, but I can handle it." This simple change in self-talk can reduce the emotional distress associated with pain.

## 5. Modeling Success Stories

Remember, one of the core principles of NLP is modeling excellence. In the context of chronic pain, this means seeking out individuals who have successfully managed their pain and learning from their strategies. By emulating their thought patterns and behaviors, you can gain valuable insights into your own pain management.

## A Journey of Self-Discovery and Healing

NLP isn't a magical cure for chronic pain, and it doesn't promise to eliminate pain entirely. However, **it equips you with a powerful set of tools and principles to regain control over your life and manage pain more effectively**. Your journey with NLP is a journey of self-discovery and healing, where you learn to navigate the intricate landscape of your mind and emotions.

By applying NLP techniques, you can reduce the emotional suffering that often accompanies chronic pain. You can develop a more positive and resilient attitude, and you can become more attuned to your body's signals and its capacity for healing. **NLP empowers you to create a life that is not defined by pain but shaped by your own desires and aspirations**.

Remember, you are not alone in your struggle with chronic pain, and there is hope. NLP offers a unique approach that can complement medical treatments and other pain management strategies. It's a journey of self-mastery that can lead to a more fulfilling, pain-free life.

As we continue this exploration of Neuro-Linguistic Programming, we will delve deeper into specific NLP techniques and applications for managing chronic pain, allowing you to gain a more comprehensive understanding of how this approach can transform your relationship with pain.

# UNVEILING THE MINDSET SHIFT

Imagine looking at your pain from a different angle, seeing it as a challenge to overcome rather than an insurmountable obstacle. The process of changing your perception of pain begins with a mindset shift. **This shift is not about denying the reality of your pain but redefining your relationship with it.** Here are some techniques that I've found invaluable in this process:

**1. Reframing Aches and Pain as a Teacher**: Instead of seeing aches and pain as an enemy stalking you day and night, consider it as a teacher instead. Pain can teach us resilience, patience, and strength. When we frame it this way, we acknowledge its existence but also transform it into a source of personal growth. By doing this, we begin to break free from the mental prison of suffering.

**2. Visualization and Mind-Body Connection**: Our minds and bodies are intrinsically connected. Using techniques like visualization, I've been able to reduce pain's intensity. I close my eyes, and in my mind I give the sensation of the pain a color – first I make the color bright and overwhelming, then I dull the color making it fade to translucent. I amy do this several times to varying degrees. The point is, this simple act of visualization sends signals to my body to relax and reduce pain.

**3. Anchoring for Pain Management**: Anchoring is a remarkable NLP technique that associates a specific trigger with a desired emotional state. I've created anchors for moments when my pain is minimal or when I experience relief. By touching a specific part of my body or using a particular word or gesture, I can trigger the anchor in times of high pain, which helps me regain a sense of control.

**4. Language and Self-Talk Transformation**: Language is a powerful tool for shaping our beliefs and perceptions. The words we choose to describe our pain can either amplify or reduce our suffering. I've become conscious of my internal dialogue and changed the way I speak to myself. Instead of using negative, disempowering words, I now choose language that acknowledges my discomfort but emphasizes my ability to handle it.

### The Power of Language in Shaping Beliefs

Let's dive deeper into the incredible power of language in shaping our beliefs and, by extension, our experience of chronic pain.

### 1. Labeling Pain

Words like "excruciating," "unbearable," or "agonizing" can intensify our pain experience. When we label pain using such words, we unconsciously reinforce the idea that it's an overwhelming force. Instead, try using neutral or even positive language. For instance, you can say, "I'm experiencing discomfort," or "I'm in a challenging moment." Some things I've occasionally said out loud "I wonder what this would feel like underwater (or in the cold, or if it were in my baby toe!) - any or all of these efforts shift the focus from the pain's intensity to your capacity to manage and or control it.

## 2. Avoid Catastrophizing

Catastrophizing is a cognitive distortion where we exaggerate the negative consequences of an event. In the context of chronic pain, it's a common thought pattern. Phrases like, "I can't handle this anymore" or "This pain will never end" feed into this distortion, making pain seem even more unbearable. Challenge these thoughts by reframing them. Replace them with statements like, "I've overcome difficult days before, and I can do it again," or "Pain is temporary, and I have strategies to manage it." I like adding a little extra umph sometimes and I'll add stuff like "*and,* I am so much more resourceful than before." Or "*and,* easy enough, I can defeat it".

## 3. Empowerment Through Language

Empowerment is about taking control of your experience. Using language that reflects your capacity to manage pain can be transformative. Phrases like "I choose to take steps to reduce and, in some ways, eliminate pain" (*note that I don't call it 'my' pain! I don't want it – so I won't own it)* or "I have the power to reduce and eliminate *this* suffering" reaffirm your ability to influence *the* pain experience. You become the protagonist in your journey, not a passive victim.

## 4. Positive Affirmations

Positive affirmations are simple, yet potent, statements that can shift your mindset. Create a list of affirmations that resonate with you and your pain management goals. For example, "I am resilient," "I am in control of *this* experience," or "I am getting better every day in every way" or "I am nurturing parts of me every day in some positive way." Repeat these affirmations regularly to reinforce your positive mindset.

## 5. Mindful Self-Compassion

Chronic pain often brings a lot of negative self-talk and self-criticism. Cultivate mindful self-compassion by treating yourself with kindness and understanding. When your pain flares up, instead of berating yourself for not coping better, offer self-compassion and guidance by saying (or writing a letter to yourself), "I'm doing the best I can, and that's enough. I get better and better every day, every day in some way, I get better and better each day" This change in language fosters self-love and resilience. *Note that I said the same thing a couple different ways – for me and my brain the more ways I can say the same thing – the more engrained it becomes.*

## My Personal Journey

I won't pretend that changing your language and perception of pain is a one-size-fits-all solution. It takes time, patience, and practice. But it's a journey worth embarking on. Let me share a little more about my personal experience with these techniques.

When I first started practicing NLP-inspired language and mindset shifts, it felt challenging. The negative self-talk had become so ingrained that I wasn't even aware of it. I'd drop something and call myself names like dummy or I'd forget my words and call myself an idiot. It was very strange to me to express vocally self-compassion! I started slow with correcting or adapting the negative talk like if out of habit I called myself a dummy for dropping something, I'd continue the sentence with something like ... "if you don't remember you are human! I love you human – keep going you got this". After a while and with daily effort, I began to catch myself using disempowering language and transform it into something more positive and affirming.

For instance, I used to say, "My pain is unbearable." Now, I say, "I'm being physically challenged, thankfully, I have a strategies to win the battle!

This shift in language not only reduces my emotional suffering but also empowers me to take proactive steps in managing the situation and reducing, and occasionally eliminating the pain.

Catastrophizing was another tough nut to crack. I often found myself spiraling into thoughts of hopelessness. But gradually, I learned to recognize these thoughts and reframe them. Instead of thinking, "This pain will never end," I began to tell myself, "Pain is temporary, and I have tools to win the battle." This simple change in perspective significantly improved my ability to endure the tough moments.

Positive affirmations and self-compassion have also played a central role in my journey. Affirmations remind me of my resilience and ability to heal, while self-compassion softens the edges of my self-criticism and reinforces my strength.

## It's a Continuous Journey

Changing your perception of chronic pain through language and mindset shifts is not a one-time endeavor. It's a continuous journey of self-discovery and transformation. Some days, you'll find it easier than others. On the difficult days, don't be too hard on yourself. Remember, you're reprogramming your brain, and that takes time.

It's essential to combine these language and mindset techniques with other pain management strategies. NLP is not a standalone solution, but it complements other approaches beautifully, making them even more effective.

By shifting your mindset and using the power of language, you can begin to reshape your relationship with chronic pain. **You can become the author of your own story, not the victim of circumstances**. With practice and perseverance, you'll find that you have more control over the pain experience than you ever thought possible.

Notably, I have found it very helpful to write myself letters, particularly on those days in which movement is limited and/or I'm having difficulty saying or thinking kindly things to or about myself.  Sitting down and putting paper to pen adds a layer of effort and sensation, enriching the experience.

Simply said remember this: You have the power to change the way you perceive and experience pain. The words you choose and the beliefs you hold are potent tools in this transformation. Embrace the power of language and the potential for a more positive, fulfilling life. You've got this!

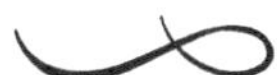

# PRACTICAL NLP EXERCISES

Living with chronic pain can feel like navigating an endless labyrinth of suffering. However, my studies and practice of Neuro-Linguistic Programming (NLP) has given me valuable tools to combat this relentless adversary. In this piece, I'll share practical NLP exercises that can help you reframe your thoughts, change the sub modalities of your pain experience, and empower you to live a life shaped by your desires and ambitions, not by pain.

## Step 1: Recognizing Negative Thought Patterns

The first step in managing chronic pain with NLP is recognizing negative thought patterns. Chronic pain often leads to a cycle of distressing thoughts, such as "I can't handle this pain" or "I'll never find relief." These patterns exacerbate suffering. By acknowledging them, you take the first step toward transformation.

## Exercise 1: Thought Journaling

1. Start by keeping a journal where you record your thoughts related to pain.

2. Whenever you notice a negative or distressing thought, write it down. Be specific.

3. Note the circumstances or triggers that led to the thought.

## Step 2: Reframe Negative Thoughts

Once you've identified negative thought patterns, the next step is to reframe them. Reframing is a powerful NLP technique that helps change the meaning of a situation or thought. Instead of seeing pain as an insurmountable obstacle, you can learn to view it as a challenge that brings growth.

## Exercise 2: Reframing Your Thoughts

1. Choose one of the negative thoughts from your thought journal.

2. Examine the thought closely and ask yourself if it serves your well-being. Does it help you cope with pain, or does it intensify your suffering?

3. Now, reframe the thought. For instance, if your thought is "I can't handle this pain," reframe it to "I am learning to manage my pain better every day."

4. Practice this new thought whenever the negative one arises. Repetition is key to solidifying this new perspective. Neurons that fire together – wire together. In other words do things enough times it becomes automatic! Habitual if you please!

## Step 3: Changing Submodalities of Pain

NLP recognizes that the sensory elements of an experience (submodalities) greatly influence how we perceive it. For chronic pain, this means that changing the submodalities can alter the intensity of the experience. Submodalities include aspects like location, color, size, and shape.

## Exercise 3: Submodalities Transformation

1. Close your eyes and focus on the sensation of pain. Take a few deep breaths to center yourself.

2. Imagine the pain as a specific color. For many, it might be red or dark.

3. Now, change the color in your mind to a calming, soothing one. Visualize it shifting from red to light blue, for instance.

4. As you do this, pay attention to how the intensity of the pain changes. For many people, the pain becomes less intense as it changes color.

5. You can also experiment with other submodalities like location (moving the pain to a different part of your body), size (making it smaller), and shape (altering it to something less threatening).

This exercise demonstrates the powerful connection between your mind and body and how you can actively influence your pain experience by altering submodalities.

## Step 4: Anchoring for Pain Management

Anchoring is an NLP technique that connects a specific trigger with a desired emotional state. By creating an anchor for pain management, you can evoke feelings of relief and relaxation in times of high pain.

## Exercise 4: Creating a Pain Management Anchor

1. Identify a moment when your pain is at a minimum or when you experience relief, however brief.

2. Choose a specific physical gesture, word, or touch that you can easily replicate in times of high pain.

3. In the low-pain state, perform this action or word while fully experiencing the relief.

4. Repeat this process several times to reinforce the association between the anchor and relief.

5. When experiencing intense pain, trigger the anchor by using the chosen gesture, word, or touch. This can help you regain a sense of control and relaxation even in the midst of suffering.

## Step 5: Language and Self-Talk Transformation

As I mentioned earlier, the language you use to describe your pain can significantly influence your experience of it. By changing your self-talk, you can empower yourself and reduce the emotional distress associated with pain.

## Exercise 5: Empowering Self-Talk

1. Start by becoming more aware of your internal dialogue. Notice the negative and disempowering words you use to describe your pain.

2. Replace these negative words with more neutral, positive, or empowering language. For example, instead of saying, "I'm in unbearable pain," you can say, "I'm experiencing discomfort, but I have the tools to manage it."

3. Create a list of positive affirmations related to pain management. For example, "I am resilient," "I can cope with pain," or "I have the power to reduce and eliminate this suffering." Repeat these affirmations regularly to reinforce your positive mindset.

## Step 6: Empowerment Through Modeling

One of the fundamental principles of NLP is modeling success. In the context of chronic pain, you can learn from individuals who have effectively managed their pain and apply their strategies to your own life.

## Exercise 6: Finding Role Models

1. Seek out stories of people who have successfully managed chronic pain. You can find these stories in books, online communities, or support groups.

2. Pay attention to their thought patterns and behaviors. What strategies do they use to cope with pain? How do they stay positive in spite of their challenges?

3. Choose one or more role models and begin to model their strategies. This might involve adopting their language, mindset, or pain management techniques.

## Step 7: Goal Setting and Aspiration

NLP is not just about managing pain; it's also about creating a life that is not defined by suffering but shaped by your desires and ambitions. This step is about setting goals and cultivating a vision for your life beyond pain.

## Exercise 7: Setting Life Goals

1. Take some time to reflect on your aspirations and desires. What are the things you'd like to achieve or experience in life?

2.  Write down these goals and aspirations. They can be related to career, personal growth, relationships, or any other aspect of life.

3.  Break these larger goals into smaller, achievable steps. This makes them more manageable and less overwhelming.

4.  Visualize yourself accomplishing these goals and living the life you desire. Use the power of your imagination to create a vivid mental picture.

5.  Whenever you face a challenging moment with pain, return to these goals and aspirations. Remind yourself of the life you are working towards. The life you will achieve as you continue to get better and better every day in every way!

**Step 8: Regular Practice and Patience**

The key to success with these NLP exercises is regular practice and patience. Like any skill, changing your perception of chronic pain takes time. Be kind to yourself on days when it's challenging and celebrate your progress along the way.

By consistently applying these NLP techniques, you can reframe your thoughts, change the sub modalities of your pain experience, and empower yourself to live a life defined by your desires, not by pain. **Chronic pain is a formidable adversary, but you have the power to transform your relationship with it and take control of your life and happiness.** Remember, you are the author of your own story, and NLP can be your guiding light on this transformative journey.

# *Hypnosis Practice*

# DEMYSTIFYING HYPNOSIS

As someone who has always been fascinated by the human mind and its vast capabilities, the world of hypnosis has been a source of intrigue and wonder for me. Over the years, I've delved deep into the subject, I studied the works from greats like Milton Erikson, James Braid (surgeon) John Milne Bramwell, Émile Coué, Dave Elman, James Esdaile, and George Estabrooks. My studies helped to separate fact from fiction, and debunk myths that often shroud the practice. Through extensive study and practice, I've come to appreciate the genuinely profound impact hypnosis can have on our lives and, how it is distinctly different from meditation.

Hypnosis, it's a word that often conjures up images of swinging pocket watches, eerie music, and mysterious figures controlling your thoughts and actions. Admittedly, I used to be one of those individuals who believed hypnosis to be little more than a stage act or a fantastical concept from movies and books. And, as we know, INFO IS POWER!

Hypnosis is often misunderstood, and many misconceptions surround it. In this section, I'll explain what hypnosis truly is, what it isn't, and how it differs from meditation. We'll also delve into the science behind hypnotic techniques and explore the value of combining Neuro-Linguistic Programming (NLP) with hypnosis to address the challenges of chronic pain.

## What Hypnosis Is and Isn't

My journey into understanding hypnosis began when I stumbled upon a documentary about its applications in various therapeutic contexts. I learned that hypnosis isn't some form of mind control or a mystical force that renders you powerless. Instead, it's a state of focused attention and heightened suggestibility.

In its essence, hypnosis is a natural and relaxed state of consciousness that most of us enter and exit several times every day. Fundamentally, it is a natural phenomenon that we all engage in regularly You've experienced it yourself when you've been so absorbed in a book or movie that you lose track of time, or when you're driving and suddenly realize you've arrived at your destination without consciously remembering the journey. These are trance-like states, similar to hypnosis.

During hypnosis, you remain in control of your thoughts and actions. You won't do anything against your will, and you can't be made to reveal your deepest secrets or commit unlawful acts. In fact, you can't be hypnotized to do something that violates your moral or ethical code.

Hypnosis involves the power of suggestion. It's like planting a seed in your mind, and if that suggestion aligns with your goals or desires, it can influence your thoughts, feelings, and behaviors in a positive way. In other words, it's a tool for self-improvement and personal growth, rather than a means of coercion.

## Hypnosis vs. Meditation

Now, before we go to much further in details, I'd like to take this opportunity to differentiate between hypnosis and meditation. Both are altered states of consciousness, but they serve distinct purposes and involve different techniques.

Meditation is a practice that seeks to cultivate mindfulness, focus, and self-awareness. It often involves quieting the mind, observing your thoughts, and achieving a state of inner calm and serenity. Meditation encourages self-reflection and is used for stress reduction, increased self-awareness, and spiritual growth.

Hypnosis, on the other hand, is a guided process that typically involves an external source (the hypnotist) providing suggestions for your subconscious mind. While meditation is generally self-directed, hypnosis relies on an external guide to lead you into a hypnotic state and provide specific suggestions tailored to your goals or challenges.

In a meditative state, you might observe your thoughts without attachment, whereas in hypnosis, you actively engage with specific suggestions meant to bring about change. While meditation is an excellent practice for general well-being, hypnosis is a more focused and goal-oriented approach.

## The Science Behind Hypnotic Techniques

To further understand hypnosis, it's crucial to explore the scientific basis of hypnotic techniques. Hypnosis is not some mystical or pseudoscientific concept; it has been studied and validated by scientific research.

During hypnosis, the brain undergoes changes in activity that are observable through various neuroimaging techniques. Functional magnetic resonance imaging (fMRI) studies have shown that during hypnosis, specific areas of the brain, including the prefrontal cortex, experience altered patterns of activation. This is indicative of a shift in consciousness and attention.

Additionally, research has demonstrated that hypnosis can be a powerful tool for pain management. Studies have revealed that under hypnosis, individuals experience changes in pain perception, reduced pain-related brain activity, and even the ability to control their response to painful stimuli. This has significant implications for those suffering from chronic pain.

## Combining NLP Techniques with Hypnosis for Chronic Pain

That said, let's address the valuable synergy of combining Neuro-Linguistic Programming (NLP) with hypnosis, particularly in the context of chronic pain management. NLP is a psychological approach that focuses on how we think, communicate, and behave. As you learned in the previous chapter, It can be used to reframe negative thought patterns, change behaviors, and enhance personal development.

Incorporating NLP into hypnosis can provide an incredibly effective approach to address chronic pain. Chronic pain often has both physical and psychological components. While interventions (like cannabis or pharmaceuticals or surgery) can address the physical aspects, the psychological factors are equally important. NLP techniques, when combined with hypnosis, can help individuals change their perception of pain, manage anxiety related to pain, and improve their overall well-being.

The process begins by identifying the specific challenges and beliefs related to pain. The NLP practitioner works with the individual to reframe negative thought patterns and beliefs about pain. For example, if someone believes, "I'll always be in pain," an NLP practitioner can help them reframe that belief into a more positive and empowering statement, such as, "I have the ability to manage my pain and improve my quality of life."

Once these beliefs are reframed, hypnosis can be used to reinforce these positive suggestions at a subconscious level. The individual is guided into a relaxed and receptive state, where they are more open to accepting and internalizing the new beliefs and behaviors.

Furthermore, NLP can provide individuals with practical tools for pain management, such as techniques for relaxation, stress reduction, and coping strategies. When these tools are combined with the power of suggestion in hypnosis, individuals can gain greater control over their pain and reduce their reliance on medication easily.

Through my journey into understanding hypnosis and the potential of combining NLP techniques, I've witnessed remarkable transformations in people's lives – including my own. Chronic pain, which can be both physically and emotionally debilitating, can be effectively managed, allowing individuals to regain a sense of control and improve their quality of life. For all intent purposes – this combination of techniques prevents chronic illness from holding your happiness hostage!

In conclusion, hypnosis is not the enigmatic, mind-controlling phenomenon portrayed in movies and stage shows. It's a state of focused attention and heightened suggestibility, which can be harnessed for self-improvement and personal growth. It differs from meditation in its guided, goal-oriented nature.

Hypnosis is grounded in scientific research, with observable changes in brain activity during hypnotic states. When combined with NLP techniques, it becomes a powerful tool for addressing chronic pain by reframing beliefs, managing stress, and empowering individuals to take control of their pain management.

My journey into understanding hypnosis opened my eyes to the incredible potential it holds for personal transformation and well-being. It's a far cry from the mysterious and sensationalized portrayal it often receives, and I encourage anyone dealing with chronic pain or seeking self-improvement to explore the world of hypnosis with an open mind and a spirit of curiosity.

# SELF HYPNOSIS

Self-hypnosis is a fascinating technique and skill that allows you to tap into the power of your subconscious mind all by yourself. It's a way to induce a state of heightened focus and suggestibility, just like hypnosis with a therapist, but you're both the guide and the subject. It takes practice and time for skill development that is worth the effort. Personally, I've found self-hypnosis is be a valuable tool for pain management, and I'm here to guide you through some practical exercises to get you started on your own journey.

**Understanding Self-Hypnosis**

Before we dive into the exercises, it's important to grasp the basics of self-hypnosis. Like traditional hypnosis, self-hypnosis involves relaxing your body and mind to access your subconscious. The key here is that you are in control, and it's a skill you can develop over time with practice.

**Self-Hypnosis Exercise for Pain Management:**

1. **Find a Quiet Space:** Start by finding a quiet, comfortable space where you won't be disturbed. Sit in a chair or lie down – whichever is more comfortable for you.

2. **Focus on Your Breathing:** Close your eyes and take a few deep breaths to calm your mind and body. Inhale deeply through your nose, allowing your lungs to fill, and then exhale slowly through your mouth. With each breath, you become more relaxed.

3. **Progressive Relaxation:** Begin by directing your attention to different parts of your body, starting from your toes and moving upwards. As you focus on each body part, imagine it becoming warm, heavy, and deeply relaxed. Feel the tension melting away.

4. **Positive Affirmations:** Now, introduce positive affirmations related to your pain management. These should be short, positive statements that reflect your goals. For instance, if you're dealing with chronic pain, affirmations like "I am in control of how I respond to this pain" or "My body knows how to heal naturally and is healing" can be powerful.

5. **Visualization:** Next, imagine a place or scenario that brings you comfort and relaxation. It might be a serene beach, a cozy cabin in the woods, or any place that feels safe and tranquil to you. Visualize the details vividly – the colors, the sounds, and the sensations. Make the image very rich.

6. **Deepening the Hypnotic State:** To deepen your self-hypnotic state, count down from 10 to 1 with each number taking you deeper into relaxation. As you count, imagine yourself descending a staircase or an elevator, feeling more and more relaxed with each step.

7. **Suggestion:** This is where you deliver your affirmations and suggestions. Repeat your positive statements while in this deep state of relaxation. Imagine them sinking into your subconscious, creating change and relief.

8. **Stay Relaxed:** Spend some time in this state, embracing the positive feelings and sensations. The more you practice, the better you'll become at maintaining this state.

9. **Return to Full Awareness:** When you're ready, slowly count from 1 to 5, with each number bringing you back to full awareness. Feel your body becoming more awake and alert.

10. **Open Your Eyes:** When you reach 5, open your eyes and take a few moments to reorient yourself to your surroundings. I often try a distraction from the state by searching for a smell I didn't notice before – Like testing to see if I can smell popcorn or pickles!

**Tips for Successful Self-Hypnosis:**

- **Consistency:** Practice self-hypnosis regularly. Like any skill, it improves with consistent effort.

- **Positive Language:** Use positive affirmations in the present tense. This helps your subconscious mind accept the suggestions more readily. And DO NOT OWN THE PAIN! Do not say things like *my* pain, because by nature humans don't want to give up or lose things they've acquired – yet, this pain is not something you want to keep, right? So don't tell your brain you own it or that its yours!

- **Belief:** Approach self-hypnosis with an open mind and a belief in its potential. Trust in your ability to influence your subconscious.

- **Be Patient:** Results may not be immediate. Keep practicing and fine-tuning your approach.

**Customizing Your Self-Hypnosis Experience:**

One of the beauties of self-hypnosis is its adaptability. You can customize it to suit your specific needs. If you find that a certain visualization or affirmation doesn't resonate with you, change it to something that does. Your self-hypnosis sessions should be tailored to your unique experiences and goals.

In conclusion, self-hypnosis is a potent tool to engage with your subconscious mind, allowing you to influence your thoughts, emotions, and even your perception of pain. By practicing the exercises outlined here and customizing them to your specific needs, you can harness the power of your mind to enhance your overall well-being and pain management. With dedication and consistency, self-hypnosis can become a valuable part of your toolkit for living a healthier and more fulfilling life.

*A Meditation Moment*

# PRACTICING MEDITATION

Meditation is a practice that has been an integral part of human history for thousands of years. Its roots trace back to ancient civilizations like India, where it was first documented in texts like the Vedas. Over time, meditation spread to other parts of the world, including China, Japan, and Tibet, each culture imbuing it with its own unique philosophies and techniques.

The historical tapestry of meditation is rich and diverse. Ancient yogis in India practiced meditation to attain enlightenment and self-realization. In China, Taoist sages meditated to find harmony with the Tao, while in Japan, Zen Buddhism introduced a unique form of meditation known for its simplicity and focus. These practices have had an enduring impact on our understanding of meditation today.

From a scientific perspective, meditation's transformative power has been a subject of great interest. Over the last few decades, numerous studies have provided valuable insights into the physical and psychological benefits of meditation. This ancient practice has shown to reduce stress, lower blood pressure, improve focus, and enhance overall well-being.

One of the key scientific components of meditation is its impact on the brain. Neuroimaging studies have revealed that regular meditation can physically change the brain by increasing grey matter density in regions associated with memory, self-awareness, and empathy. This neurological plasticity allows individuals to rewire their thought patterns and responses to stress, making it an essential tool in managing mental health.

## The Value and Benefits of a Regular Meditation Practice

The benefits of meditation are not limited to a select few. They are accessible to anyone willing to commit to a regular practice. So, what can you expect to gain from meditation?

1. **Stress Reduction**: In today's fast-paced world, stress is a common companion. Meditation acts as a soothing balm for your mind. It helps you regulate stress levels and improve your ability to manage life's daily challenges.

2. **Enhanced Emotional Well-Being**: Regular meditation cultivates emotional resilience and helps you develop a greater sense of emotional balance. It encourages self-awareness and mindfulness, allowing you to respond more skillfully to emotional challenges.

3. **Improved Concentration and Cognitive Function**: Meditation enhances your ability to concentrate and boosts cognitive functions such as memory and problem-solving. This makes it an excellent tool for students, professionals, and anyone seeking to enhance their mental acuity.

4. **Better Sleep**: Insomnia and sleep-related issues are common problems in today's society. Meditation can lead to better sleep patterns and improved sleep quality, helping you wake up feeling refreshed and energized.

5. **Pain Management**: Meditation has been increasingly recognized as an effective complementary therapy for pain management. It can alleviate chronic pain by reducing the perception of pain and increasing pain tolerance. This is where the synergy between meditation and cannabis becomes particularly interesting.

## Meditation and Cannabis for Chronic Pain Relief

Chronic pain can be an unrelenting, debilitating condition that affects millions of people worldwide. Traditional pain management options, such as opioids, often come with a host of adverse effects and can lead to addiction. In this context, meditation and cannabis can offer a holistic, non-pharmaceutical approach to pain relief.

1. **Meditation and Pain Management**: The practice of meditation can reduce the perception of pain by altering the way your brain processes it. By focusing your mind and cultivating mindfulness during meditation, you can increase your pain tolerance and reduce the distress associated with chronic pain. This mind-body connection is particularly useful in managing pain conditions such as arthritis, fibromyalgia, and migraines.

2. **Cannabis and Pain Relief**: Cannabis, on the other hand, contains compounds called cannabinoids, most notably tetrahydrocannabinol (THC) and cannabidiol (CBD), which have shown great promise in managing chronic pain. THC is known for its psychoactive effects and its ability to mitigate pain, while CBD is non-psychoactive and helps reduce inflammation and anxiety, often associated with chronic pain.

When combined with meditation, the effects of cannabis on pain can be amplified. Meditation can help you focus your mind, making it easier to harness the potential of these cannabinoids. As you meditate, you become more attuned to your body and its sensations, allowing you to better understand how cannabis influences your pain perception.

3. **The Entourage Effect**: Some researchers believe that there is a synergistic effect between meditation and cannabis, known as the "entourage effect." This suggests that combining meditation with cannabis may lead to greater pain relief than using either method alone. By calming your mind and body through meditation, you can enhance the effectiveness of the cannabinoids in reducing pain.

4. **Reduced Opioid Dependency**: The opioid crisis has drawn attention to the need for alternative pain management strategies. For those struggling with opioid addiction due to chronic pain, combining meditation and cannabis may offer a way to reduce reliance on opioids. While this approach may not be suitable for everyone, it's certainly worth exploring with the guidance of healthcare professionals.

## A Holistic Approach to Pain Management

It's important to emphasize that the combination of meditation and cannabis for chronic pain management should be approached with care and responsibility. It's crucial to consult with a medical professional, especially when considering cannabis use, to ensure it's appropriate for your condition and to address potential risks or interactions with other medications.

In addition to pain relief, this holistic approach can also offer a range of other benefits. It can help improve sleep, reduce stress and anxiety, and promote a sense of well-being. Moreover, it aligns with the growing movement toward more natural and integrative healthcare options.

In conclusion, the journey of meditation is a deeply personal one. It is a path to self-discovery, healing, and peace. The ancient wisdom of meditation, combined with the potential healing properties of cannabis, offers hope and relief to those who suffer from chronic pain. By exploring this holistic approach, you have the opportunity to unlock the power of your mind and the natural gifts of the earth, enhancing your overall quality of life. So, why not give it a try? After all, the path to healing and self-discovery might just be a quiet, meditative moment away.

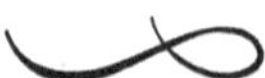

# THE PATH TO INNER PEACE

As someone who has personally experienced the transformative power of meditation, I'd like to share my journey with you and guide you through the steps to begin your own meditation practice.

**Getting Started with Meditation**

1. **Choose a Comfortable Space**: Find a quiet and comfortable spot where you won't be disturbed. Whether it's a cozy corner in your home or a peaceful park, the location is key to your meditation practice.

2. **Comfortable Posture**: Sit down with your back straight, either on a cushion or a chair. You can also lie down if that's more comfortable, but be cautious not to fall asleep. Rest your hands on your lap or knees. Close your eyes gently.

3. **Focus on Your Breath**: Start by taking a few deep breaths, inhaling through your nose and exhaling through your mouth. After a few deep breaths, let your breath return to its natural rhythm. Pay close attention to the sensation of your breath as it moves in and out of your body. The rising and falling of your chest or the coolness of the air entering your nostrils are excellent focal points.

4. **Mindfulness of the Body**: Begin a body scan, starting at the top of your head and slowly moving your awareness down to your toes. As you do this, let go of any tension you may be holding. If you encounter areas of pain or discomfort, breathe into them. Imagine your breath soothing and healing these areas.

5. **Let Thoughts Flow**: Your mind will naturally wander. This is completely normal. When you notice your mind drifting to other thoughts, acknowledge them without judgment and gently guide your focus back to your breath or the body scan.

6. **Set a Timer**: To begin, consider setting a timer for 10-15 minutes. As you become more comfortable with meditation, you can extend the duration as you see fit.

7. **Meditation Apps and Guided Sessions**: If you're just starting, there are various meditation apps and guided sessions available that can help you stay on track and provide you with additional tips and techniques.

## Practical Exercises for Pain Management

Now, let's explore practical exercises to help manage chronic pain through meditation.

1. **Breath Focus for Pain Relief**:

- As you sit or lie down in your meditation posture, bring your attention to the area of pain in your body.

- Breathe gently and consciously into that area, visualizing your breath as a soothing, healing energy.

- As you exhale, imagine releasing tension and pain from the area. Focus on the sensation of warmth and relief with each breath.

- Continue this for a few minutes, then gradually return your awareness to your entire body, noticing how the pain has subsided.

2. **Body Scan for Pain Relief**:

- Begin the body scan as described earlier, but this time, focus on the specific area where you experience pain.

- When you reach the area of pain, pause and breathe into it. Visualize your breath as a healing light, radiating warmth and comfort.

- Imagine the pain dissipating with each breath, allowing relaxation and relief to take its place.

- Slowly continue the body scan, paying extra attention to areas of pain and discomfort, offering your breath as a source of comfort and release.

3. **Mindful Pain Observation**:

- Instead of trying to eliminate the pain, sit with it. Allow yourself to fully observe and acknowledge the sensations without judgment.

- Notice how the pain feels – its quality, intensity, and any changes that occur. It may not make the pain disappear, but it can reduce the emotional suffering that often accompanies it.

- Be patient and kind to yourself. Chronic pain can be challenging, but by mindfully observing it, you may find it more manageable over time.

4. **Loving-Kindness Meditation for Pain**:

- This practice involves sending positive and loving energy to yourself and others. It can be particularly helpful for those struggling with pain.

- Sit comfortably, close your eyes, and focus on your breath for a few minutes.

- When you're ready, imagine a warm, loving light radiating from your heart and enveloping your entire body.

- As you breathe in and out, silently repeat phrases like "May I be free from suffering. May I be healthy. May I live with ease." Then extend these wishes to others who may be experiencing pain or hardship.

These exercises are meant to be practiced regularly, ideally daily. With time and dedication, you can develop the skills to manage chronic pain more effectively and improve your overall quality of life. Remember, meditation is a journey, and the benefits may not always be immediate. Be patient with yourself, and you'll likely discover a sense of peace and pain relief that you never thought possible.

Meditation, when combined with mindfulness and compassion, can lead to a profound shift in how we perceive and cope with chronic pain. By incorporating these practices into your daily routine, you have the opportunity to cultivate a sense of inner peace, reduce suffering, and discover a path to healing that is entirely your own.

# *Reclaiming Health, Wellness & Happiness*

# MY STORY IN SHORT

Reclaiming My Life: Battling Chronic Pain and Finding Healing

In my early 30s, I never imagined that I would be thrust into a battle against an invisible enemy that would alter the course of my life. As I reflect on my journey, I realize that my experiences have been a rollercoaster ride of challenges, successes, and setbacks. It all began when I was a budding entrepreneur, running a virtual assistance business during a time when the internet was still a novelty to many. I had two young children to care for, lived in an old farmhouse 20 minutes from town, and to top it all off, I had just embarked on a new romantic relationship. Life seemed full of possibilities, but chronic pain, fatigue, and denial was about to change everything.

The first inklings of trouble emerged as nagging aches and inexplicable fatigue. I attributed these symptoms to the demanding nature of my entrepreneurial endeavors, juggling clients, and managing a household and social life. Little did I know that these discomforts would snowball into a relentless and debilitating condition that would consume my life for years.

One of the most significant challenges I faced was the gradual erosion of my physical abilities. Simple tasks became arduous, and the pain was a constant companion. I recall the days when I could no longer carry my a simple cup of coffee with confidence, a heart-wrenching realization for any person with a sense of independence. The frustration and sadness were overwhelming, and my inability to be the "go-getter" kind of person I wanted to be weighed heavily on my heart and mind.

The journey to a diagnosis was long and arduous. Multiple doctors' visits, endless blood tests, and an assortment of pharmaceutical treatments followed. Each attempt to alleviate the pain seemed like a roll of the dice, with no guaranteed outcome. The uncertainty of not knowing the cause of my suffering was emotionally draining, and it seemed like I was stuck in a never-ending loop of trial and error.

After several years of this relentless pain and confusion, I received a diagnosis that would ultimately shape the course of my battle – fibromyalgia and (inconclusive) multiple sclerosis. Alongside this, there were other conditions (ulcerative colitis, IBS, vitamin/mineral deficiencies) and co-morbidities that further complicated my situation. The diagnosis was a double-edged sword. On one hand, it provided a name for the invisible monster that had taken over my life, validating my experiences. On the other hand, it was a harsh reminder that this was a chronic condition, with no known cure.

The pharmaceutical haze that enveloped my life for the next seven to ten years is a period I look back on with mixed feelings. These drugs, prescribed in an attempt to manage my pain and related symptoms, had side effects that often felt worse than the condition they were meant to treat. I was in a constant state of grogginess, bedridden for days on end and reliant on an electric wheelchair to move around. While they provided temporary relief, I felt like a shadow of my former self.

During this period, I was not only battling physical pain but also grappling with the emotional toll it took on me and those around me. The relationships I had cherished were strained as my health issues took center stage. My new romantic relationship faced countless tests, as my partner had to come to terms with the reality of being in a relationship with someone who was often bedridden or wheelchair-bound. It required an extraordinary level of understanding, patience, and compassion on their part.

As an entrepreneur, the impact of my health struggles on my business was profound. I watched as clients slowly drifted away, unable to rely on my services consistently. The dream I had nurtured of a flourishing virtual assistance business started to crumble. I found myself at a crossroads, faced with the daunting prospect of letting go of my entrepreneurial aspirations and seeking alternative means of income.

Throughout this ordeal, one of the most critical lessons I learned was the importance of self-advocacy. I had to become my own advocate within the complex and often frustrating healthcare system. I had to educate myself about fibromyalgia and its management, and I had to persistently seek out doctors who were willing to listen and work with me. This process of self-advocacy was empowering, and it allowed me to take back some control over my life.

Amid the relentless trials, there were also moments of resilience and hope. I discovered the therapeutic potential of alternative approaches that would eventually lead me out of the pharmaceutical fog that had enveloped me for so long. It was a three-pronged strategy: cannabis, neuro-linguistic programming (NLP), and hypnosis.

Cannabis was a game-changer. I had initially been skeptical, given the stigma surrounding it, but I was desperate for relief. It turned out to be a lifeline, providing not just pain relief but also improved sleep and an overall sense of well-being. It allowed me to reduce my reliance on pharmaceutical drugs, which had been holding me hostage for far too long.

Neuro-Linguistic Programming (NLP) and hypnosis were the psychological components of my strategy. They helped me reframe my mindset and beliefs about pain, providing me with the mental tools I needed to cope. These techniques taught me to shift my focus from pain to possibilities, from limitations to empowerment. I gradually let go of the identity of a chronic pain sufferer and embraced the possibility of a healthier, happier life. I was learning that I could be "differently-abled" vs disabled.

The transition from being bedridden or wheelchair-bound to being able to walk daily, hike weekly, and even dance with my grandchildren was a gradual but remarkable transformation. It was not a linear path, and there were setbacks along the way. There were days when pain flared up, reminding me of its presence. But the difference was that I now had a set of tools at my disposal to manage those setbacks and continue on my path to recovery.

The support of my partner was instrumental during this time. He stood by me through every step of my journey, offering unwavering support and encouragement. His belief in my ability to overcome the odds and regain my life was a constant source of motivation.

As I reach my mid-fifties, I can proudly say that I am pharmaceutical-free and rarely, if ever, stuck in bed. The chronic pain that once held me hostage has been replaced by a renewed sense of power, hope and purpose. My journey has been nothing short of a miracle, made possible by the therapeutic combination of cannabis, NLP, and hypnosis – the pillars of my Battle Strategy.

Cannabis, with its pain-relieving properties, played a significant role in rescuing me from consuming copious amounts of painkillers. It allowed me to manage my pain without the debilitating side effects of pharmaceutical drugs. It was a ray of sunshine that pierced through the dark clouds of that pain created, and I found myself able to engage in activities in spite of the constant bouts of pain I experienced.

When I chose to eliminate the 93 pills I took each day, along with the fentanyl patch I had been using for years – I engaged in very risky behaviour by ending my use of pharmaceuticals abruptly – cold turkey as some would say, and I got lucky!  The detox did not kill me much to my surprise, the surprise of my doctor and pharmacist. That said, it damn near did and SO IF YOU ARE TAKING PHARMACEUTICAL MEDICATIONS – work with your doctor to reduce and eliminate, the damage done from the risks I took could have been avoided and my road to recovery may have been easier.

I continued using cannabis in a variety of ways from infusing nearly every meal I consumed to wrapping my body in infused muslin wraps. I smoked and vaped as often as I pleased or felt the need, and I began to research this miraculous plant. Learning all the health and wellness benefits that can be gleaned and the science of why!

Notably however, NLP and hypnosis, were the keys to unlocking my potential for self healing. These techniques taught me to reframe my thoughts and beliefs about pain, allowing me to regain control over my life. The power of the mind is a force to be reckoned with, and I harnessed it to break free from the chains of pain and illness that held my health, wellness, and happiness hostage.

My daily routine now includes walking, something I had once considered a distant dream. I lace up my shoes and venture out into the world with Wookiee my faithful furry companion, grateful for the simple act of putting one foot in front of the other. Weekly hikes in the great outdoors have become a cherished ritual, connecting me with nature and providing a sense of peace and tranquility that I had long been deprived of.

The most delightful transformation of all has been my return to the joyful play and goofy dancing I so enjoyed once with my children. I can now twirl, move, and groove with abandon, reveling in the joy and goofiness with my grandchildren. Dancing is not just an expression of physical freedom but also a celebration of the happiness that was held hostage by pain for too long. It is a testament to the resilience of the human spirit and the power of determination.

Through my journey, I have gleaned several insights that have guided me in my battle against chronic pain. The first and most crucial lesson is the importance of self-advocacy. It's imperative to be an active participant in your healthcare journey, to seek out the information and support you need, and to find healthcare providers who are willing to work with you as a partner in your healing process.

Another key insight is the value of alternative approaches to pain management. While pharmaceutical drugs may provide relief, they often come with a host of side effects that can be as debilitating as the condition itself. Exploring alternative therapies, like cannabis, NLP, and hypnosis, can be a game-changer in one's battle against chronic pain – I'm happy that you've taken a step in the same direction

Furthermore, it's essential to acknowledge the emotional toll that chronic pain can take. It's not just physical suffering; it's a challenge to one's mental and emotional well-being. Finding ways to cope, whether through therapy, support groups, or self-help techniques, can be a lifeline in the darkest of times.

My journey has also reinforced the importance of a strong support system. Whether it's the unwavering support of a partner, the understanding of friends and family, or the camaraderie of fellow chronic pain warriors, having a network of people who believe in you and your ability to heal is invaluable.

As I look back on my battles with chronic pain, I can't help but be grateful for the strength it has brought out in me. It was a journey filled with challenges, but it was also a journey of self-discovery, resilience, and, ultimately, triumph. **I am no longer defined by my pain; I am defined by my ability to overcome it.**

If I could offer one piece of advice to anyone facing a similar battle, it would be this: Never give up. There may be moments when the pain feels insurmountable, when the weight of it all threatens to crush your spirit. But within you lies the power to rise above it, to reclaim your health, wellness, and happiness.

My story is a testament to the fact that even in the darkest of times, there is hope. With the right tools, the support of loved ones, and an unwavering belief in your own resilience, you can overcome the most formidable challenges. Chronic pain may be a formidable foe, but with the right battle strategy, you can emerge victorious.

# *Empowerment & Integration*

# THE FIRST LINE OF DEFENSE

**The Info-Is-Power Series promotes the approach of using Cannabis, Neuro-Linguistic Programming, and Hypnosis as the pillars to create a Battle Strategy – In this title, A Battle Strategy to Combat Chronic Pain**

Chronic pain can be a debilitating condition, and a multi-faceted approach to manage it is often the most effective. Combining cannabis with Neuro-Linguistic Programming (NLP) and hypnosis, along with adopting a healthy lifestyle, can provide a comprehensive strategy for addressing chronic pain. This approach aims to alleviate pain, enhance psychological well-being, and promote overall health.

Additionally, understanding popular cannabis strains, such as Kosher Kush and Granddaddy Purple, will aid in choosing the most appropriate one for pain management.

**1. Cannabis for Chronic Pain Management:** Cannabis has been recognized for its therapeutic benefits in managing chronic pain. Different strains have varying profiles of cannabinoids and terpenes, making them suitable for different types of pain. Here are five popular strains, each with its own unique profile:

- **Kosher Kush:**

    - Strain Profile: Indica-dominant hybrid

    - Cannabinoids: High THC, low CBD

    - Terpenes: Myrcene, caryophyllene

    - Effect: Deep relaxation, pain relief, and muscle relaxation

- **Granddaddy Purple:**

    - Strain Profile: Indica

    - Cannabinoids: High THC, moderate CBD

    - Terpenes: Myrcene, pinene

    - Effect: Pain relief, relaxation, and sleep aid

- **Blue Dream:**

    - Strain Profile: Sativa-dominant hybrid

    - Cannabinoids: Balanced THC and CBD

    - Terpenes: Limonene, myrcene

    - Effect: Euphoria, pain relief, and mood elevation

- **Harlequin:**

- Strain Profile: Sativa-dominant hybrid

- Cannabinoids: High CBD, low THC

- Terpenes: Terpinolene, myrcene

- Effect: Pain relief, relaxation, without the psychoactive "high"

- **ACDC:**

  - Strain Profile: Sativa-dominant hybrid

  - Cannabinoids: High CBD, low THC

  - Terpenes: Myrcene, pinene

  - Effect: Pain relief, relaxation, and mental clarity

Notably, *CBGTV's BudBreak* is an excellent resource for exploring these strains and more, with detailed information on their therapeutic benefits and effects. Available on Amazon - scan the QR CODE.

## 2. Combining Cannabis with NLP and Hypnosis:

- **Neuro-Linguistic Programming (NLP):** NLP techniques can help reframe negative thought patterns associated with pain. Practicing NLP with a certified practitioner can aid in building a positive mindset. And using the techniques laid out in the pages of this book, learning this skill independently is more than possible.

- **Hypnosis:** Hypnotherapy can be used to manage pain perception and alleviate anxiety. A trained hypnotherapist can guide you through sessions to reduce pain sensitivity. Developing **Self-Hypnosis** skills is very empowering.

## 3. Using Cannabis in Various Forms:

- **Topical Solutions:** Cannabis-infused creams, balms, and oils can be applied directly to the affected area for localized pain relief.

- **Edibles:** Explore cannabis-infused edibles, such as gummies or chocolates, for longer-lasting pain relief. Always start with a low dose and wait for effects to avoid overconsumption.

- **Medicated Menu:** Incorporate cannabis into your diet with carefully dosed recipes. This can provide a consistent way to manage pain while enjoying food.

- **Smoking or Vaping:** Smoking or vaping cannabis offers rapid pain relief. Choose strains according to your preference and needs.

Remember that it's crucial to consult with a professional before starting any new treatment, especially if you're using cannabis for the first time. Or you wish to use it specifically for pain management. They can provide guidance on dosages, potential interactions with other medications, and monitor your progress.

Incorporating cannabis, NLP, and hypnosis into your pain management strategy, alongside a healthy lifestyle, can significantly improve your quality of life and provide long-term relief from chronic pain.

## 4. Healthy Lifestyle and Habits:

- **Exercise:** Incorporate regular, low-impact physical activity, such as yoga, swimming, or walking, to improve flexibility and reduce pain.

- **Diet:** Maintain a balanced diet rich in anti-inflammatory foods like fruits, vegetables, and omega-3 fatty acids. Consider consulting a nutritionist.

- **Meditation and Relaxation:** Practice mindfulness and deep breathing exercises to reduce stress and enhance your pain coping mechanisms.

- **Adequate Sleep:** Prioritize quality sleep to support pain management and overall well-being.

- **Hydration:** Stay well-hydrated to support bodily functions and medication effectiveness.

This strategy combines the benefits of cannabis with psychological and lifestyle approaches to effectively combat chronic pain.

The following is a typical day of applying the above battle strategy – to share with you an example to follow.

Creating a typical day routine to combat chronic aches and pains, incorporating the elements of the battle strategy, can significantly improve your quality of life. Here's a sample daily routine:

**Morning:**

1. **NLP "Happy" Anchor:** Start your day with a positive mindset. Activate your NLP "happy" anchor by taking a few moments to recall a joyful memory or visualize a happy future. This sets a positive tone for the day.

2. **Stretch Routine:** Begin with a gentle stretching routine to wake up your muscles and improve flexibility. Focus on areas prone to pain or stiffness, such as the back, neck, and joints. Incorporate deep breathing to enhance relaxation.

3. **Hydrate:** Drink a glass of water to hydrate your body and kickstart your organs. Staying hydrated is essential for overall well-being.

4. **Breakfast Smoothie:** Prepare a nutritious smoothie using a recipe from the book "Cooking with Cannabis." You can infuse it with raw cannabis (for a non-psychoactive option) or choose a CBD or THC oil depending on your pain management needs. Ensure the smoothie includes anti-inflammatory ingredients like berries, leafy greens, and healthy fats like avocado.

**Midday:**

5. **Cannabis for Pain Relief:** If you experience pain flare-ups during the day, use cannabis as needed in a way that suits your preferences and pain level.

   - Topical solutions can be applied for localized relief, or you can consume edibles or use inhalation methods for faster-acting relief.

   - Remember to consult CBGTV's BudBreak for strain recommendations. Available on Amazon in the INFO IS POWER Series.

6. **Healthy Habits:** Throughout the day, maintain healthy habits. Ensure you're moving and stretching regularly, staying hydrated, and practicing stress management techniques as needed. Smile at a stranger and add a "new nice habit" 😊

## Evening:

7. **Dinner:** Enjoy a well-balanced dinner that includes anti-inflammatory foods. Opt for lean proteins, vegetables, and whole grains to support your overall health.

8. **Meditation for Relaxation:** Before bedtime, engage in a guided meditation session to promote relaxation and improve sleep quality. This meditation can also incorporate elements of hypnotherapy, helping you reframe your perception of pain and stress.

## Additional Tips:

- **Regular Monitoring:** Keep a pain journal to track your pain levels and the effectiveness of your pain management strategies. Adjust your cannabis dosage or strain as needed.

- **Consult Professionals:** Regularly consult with healthcare professionals, including a cannabis specialist, physical therapist, and a certified NLP practitioner, to ensure your pain management strategy remains effective and safe.

- **Mind-Body Practices:** Throughout the day, practice mindfulness and relaxation techniques to keep stress at bay, which can exacerbate pain.

- **Quality Sleep:** Prioritize a good night's sleep by maintaining a consistent sleep schedule and creating a comfortable sleep environment.

- **Exercise:** Incorporate low-impact exercises as part of your daily routine to maintain flexibility and strengthen your body.

Remember, every individual's needs and responses to treatments may vary, so tailor this routine to your specific requirements and consult with professionals for personalized guidance. With dedication and a comprehensive strategy like this, you can effectively manage and change chronic pain to occasional flare-ups, even eliminating some types of pain, and improve your overall well-being.

# *Final words and wishes*

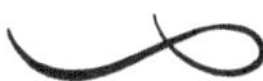

# CONCLUDING COMMENTS

As I sit here, reflecting on the journey we've taken through the pages of "Combat Chronic Pain Using Cannabis, NLP, and Hypnosis," I'm overwhelmed by a sense of hope and empowerment. This book has been more than just words on paper; it has been a journey of discovery, self-healing, and the realization that the power to combat chronic pain is within the reach of each and every one of us.

Chronic pain is an unwelcome guest that has plagued countless lives. It's not just a physical ailment; it's a relentless shadow that can dim the brightest of days. Throughout this book, we've explored various tools and techniques to reclaim our lives from the clutches of pain. But, in this concluding chapter, I want to emphasize the most crucial message of all: the power to combat chronic pain resides within us.

I understand that chronic pain is a complex and deeply personal experience. It varies in intensity, duration, and origin. Some of us might be dealing with the constant throbbing of a migraine, the burning sensation of neuropathic pain, or the relentless ache of arthritis. Others might be grappling with emotional pain, such as the grief of losing a loved one or the despair of a chronic illness. No matter the source of your pain, the first step towards healing is the understanding that you have the power to influence it.

One of the key messages of this book has been the potential of cannabis as a powerful tool in the battle against chronic pain. Cannabis, with its various compounds like CBD and THC, has shown remarkable promise in alleviating pain, reducing inflammation, and improving the overall quality of life for many individuals. However, the responsible and informed use of cannabis is vital. Consultation with a medical professional and adherence to local laws and regulations is a must.

NLP (Neuro-Linguistic Programming) and hypnosis are two other tools in our arsenal against pain. These techniques empower us to reprogram our thought patterns, beliefs, and behaviors. By doing so, we can change the way we perceive and react to pain. NLP and hypnosis provide us with the ability to tap into the immense power of our subconscious mind. We can cultivate a positive mindset and transform our pain into a catalyst for personal growth and resilience.

In this concluding chapter, I want to share a few guiding principles that can help you on your journey to combat chronic pain:

1. **Believe in Your Power**: First and foremost, believe in your ability to influence your pain. The mind-body connection is a potent force, and your belief in your own strength is a fundamental building block of healing.

2. **Seek Professional Guidance**: Consult with medical professionals and experts who can guide you in your journey. They can provide you with insights into the best treatments,

including the responsible use of cannabis, and they can help you tailor NLP and hypnosis techniques to your specific needs.

3. **Embrace Holistic Healing**: Chronic pain often has physical, emotional, and psychological dimensions. To address it effectively, embrace a holistic approach. This might include physical therapy, counseling, meditation, and a healthy lifestyle. Holistic healing recognizes the interconnectedness of our physical and mental well-being.

4. **Practice Mindfulness**: Mindfulness is the practice of being fully present in the moment. It's a powerful tool for managing chronic pain. By focusing on the now, you can reduce anxiety and stress, which are known to exacerbate pain. Regular mindfulness practice can also enhance your ability to endure pain with grace.

5. **Cultivate Resilience**: Chronic pain is a formidable adversary, but you are even more formidable. Use your pain as a catalyst for personal growth and resilience. Embrace the challenges it presents, and let them shape you into a stronger, more compassionate, and wiser individual.

6. **Connect with Others**: You're not alone in your battle against chronic pain. Reach out to support groups and connect with individuals who understand your struggle. Sharing your experiences and learning from others can be a source of comfort and valuable insights.

7. **Celebrate Small Wins**: The path to healing is not always linear, and there will be setbacks. But remember, each small victory is a step forward. Celebrate these wins, no matter how insignificant they might seem. They are proof of your progress.

8. **Visualize a Pain-Free Future**: NLP and hypnosis offer powerful visualization techniques. Take time each day to visualize a future where pain is no longer the central figure in your life. The mind is a potent tool, and positive visualization can influence your reality.

In conclusion, the journey to combat chronic pain is a deeply personal and unique one. This book has been a roadmap, but you are the driver. You hold the wheel, and you determine the direction of your journey. The power to combat chronic pain resides within you, waiting to be awakened.

I want to leave you with a final message of hope and empowerment. No matter how long you've been in the clutches of chronic pain, no matter how many tears you've shed, and no matter how many moments of despair you've endured, remember that you are more powerful than your pain. You are not defined by your pain; you are defined by your courage, resilience, and your unyielding spirit.

Take the knowledge and tools from this book and use them as a sword and shield in your battle. You are a warrior, and your battlefield is your life. In the face of chronic pain, you have the capacity to thrive, not just survive. You can emerge from this battle stronger, more compassionate, and with a deep understanding of the extraordinary power that resides within you.

Embrace this journey with an open heart and an unwavering spirit. The pain might linger, but it doesn't have to rule your life. You are the author of your story, and you have the power to write a narrative of resilience, triumph, and ultimately, healing. Chronic pain is just one chapter; it's not the whole book.

So, go forth with hope in your heart, and let the empowerment of self-discovery be your guiding star. Your journey to combat chronic pain is within your reach, and it begins with the belief that you have the power to heal and the strength to thrive once more. Your future is a canvas waiting for your brushstrokes; paint it with the colors of joy, health, and an enduring sense of well-being.

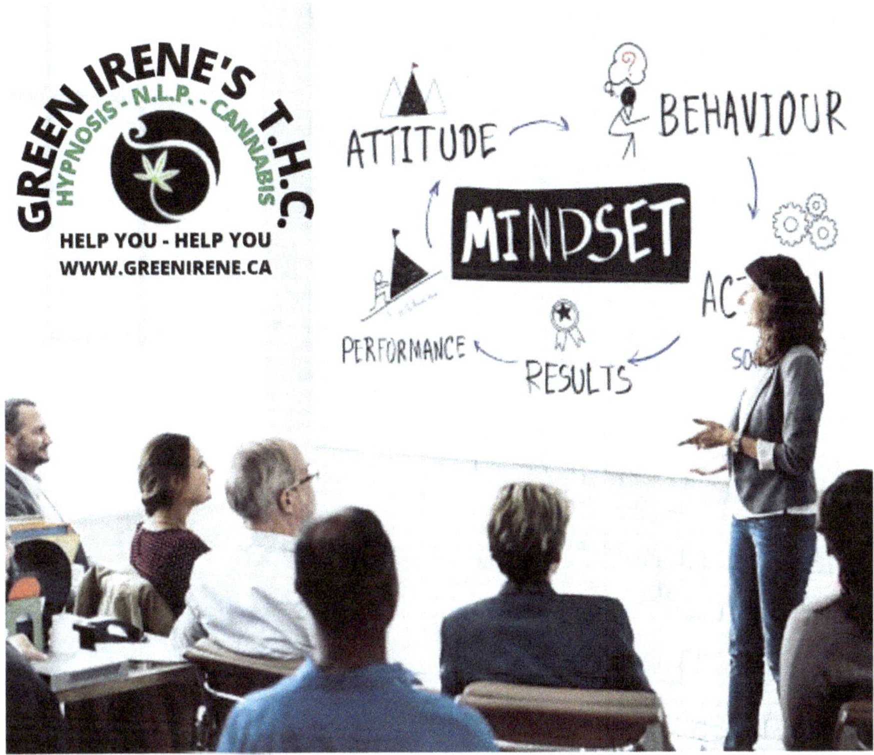

# *More Information &*
# *Resources*

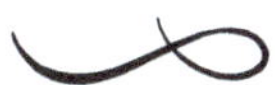

# ABOUT THE AUTHOR: GREEN IRENE AKA IRENE A YORK

Struggling with chronic conditions like fibromyalgia, digestive issues, or sleep challenges? Seeking mental well-being and positive life transformation?

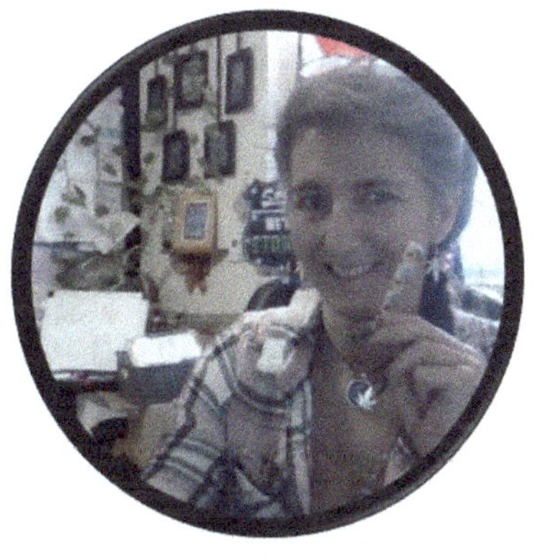

Look no further, because Irene A York, known as Green Irene, is your guiding light in the realm of alternative medicine and holistic health. With over a decade of experience and a passion for empowering others to take control of their well-being, Irene has emerged as a pioneer in her field.

What Makes Green Irene Unique? Irene's journey to becoming a trusted figure in "H E A L T H Y S E L F" holistic healing is defined by her rich life experiences and unwavering commitment to research. After spending a decade or so in a bed or a wheelchair, existing in a pharmaceutical haze, she ELEVATED & EDUCATED herself back to life using Cannabis,

NLP, and Hypnosis. Living pharmaceutically free for more than a decade now! She has full mobility and lives an active lifestyle. She has dedicated herself to helping individuals like you not just manage but thrive despite chronic conditions. Irene knows that healing is a journey, and from her own experiences, she has developed a powerful approach that combines three pillars, shared in every book of the Info Is Power Series:

1. **Cannabis for Healing**: Irene believes in the therapeutic potential of cannabis and has harnessed its power to alleviate pain, reduce inflammation, and enhance overall well-being.

2. **Hypnosis for Mental Well-being**: Mental health is a cornerstone of her approach. Through hypnosis, Irene empowers you to conquer your fears, manage stress, and embrace a more positive outlook on life.

3. **NLP (Neuro-Linguistic Programming) for Transformation**: Irene utilizes the incredible capabilities of NLP to help you create lasting change in your life, crafting a brighter tomorrow filled with hope.

📺 **Irene's Online Programs and TV Shows** Irene A York is not just a practitioner but also a prolific creator of informative content. She has produced and hosted several online programs, including "Fight Fibromyalgia," "Battle Strategies," "Cannabis & Creative Visualizations," and "A Bud Break on CBGTV." Her shows provide practical insights and inspiration for those seeking healing and transformation.

📡 **RogersTV's "Cannabis Conversations"** Irene's dedication to sharing knowledge extends to the community. She researched, hosted, and co-produced the enlightening "Cannabis Conversations" program on RogersTV, shedding light on the potential of cannabis for well-being.

📚 **"Info Is Power" Series** Irene is also a prolific author, publishing several books a year as part of the "Info Is Power" series of guides and journals. Her written works are invaluable resources for anyone seeking guidance and understanding on their journey to holistic health.

🎤 **Book Signings and Speaking Engagements** Irene A York is available to connect with her readers and followers. You can meet her in person at book signings or invite her as a guest speaker for your event, where she will share her wealth of knowledge and insights.

🌐 **Connect with Irene A York, aka Green Irene** For those seeking Irene's guidance and wisdom, reach out via her website at www.greenirene.ca. In a world where social media trends come and go, Irene remains steadfast in her commitment to helping you achieve optimal health and well-being. Alternatively, you can contact her through email at info@greenirene.ca or schedule a virtual session to embark on your journey toward a healthier, happier, and more fulfilling life.

Irene A York, aka Green Irene, is not just a pioneer; she is your partner on the path to holistic health and wellness. **HELP YOU – HELP YOU...** Take the first step towards a brighter future and contact Irene today!

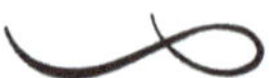

# THE INFO IS POWER SERIES

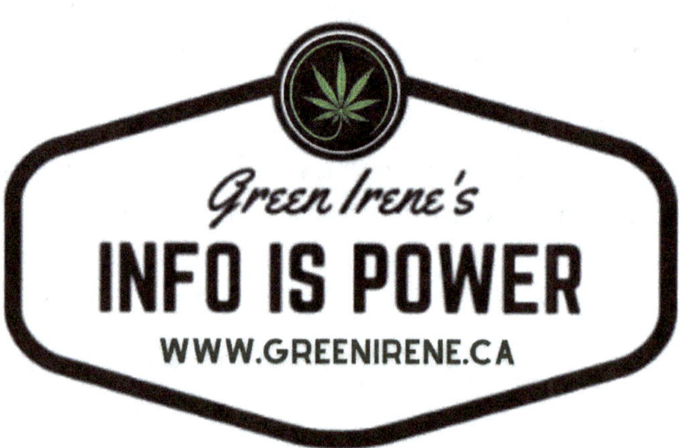


In the labyrinth of life's challenges, chronic aches and pains, illness, and disease can often make us feel powerless. The ever-present struggle to regain control over our well-being can be a daunting journey, filled with uncertainty and frustration. However, there's a guiding light in the form of the "Info is Power" series, penned and published by the remarkable Green Irene, also known as Irene A. York. These insightful books and guides serve as indispensable tools, enabling patients to reclaim the reins of their lives and transform adversity into triumph. With a friendly tone and an unwavering commitment to empower individuals in the face of health challenges, this series offers a plethora of valuable strategies that employ cannabis, neuro-linguistic programming (NLP), and hypnosis to combat a range of health and wellness hurdles.

In today's age, information is synonymous with power, and Irene A. York understands the transformative potential it holds. Through her "Info is Power" series, she provides an extensive library of resources that equip readers with the knowledge and strategies necessary to take charge of their health and well-being. Whether you are grappling with arthritis, digestive issues, chronic pain, depression, or sleep disturbances, these books offer a beacon of hope, guiding you towards a healthier, happier life.

The "Info is Power" series comprises a range of titles, each focusing on specific health and wellness challenges. These meticulously crafted books serve as personalized battle strategies, addressing issues through unique and effective approaches. The series includes titles such as "Attack Arthritis," "Battle Beastly Bowels," "Combat Chronic Pain," "Cookin' with Cannabis," "CBGTV's Bud Break Strain Reviews," "Cannabis Consumption Journals," "Defeat Depression Drama," "Tincture Time," "Strategic Sleep Solutions," and more.

One of the standout features of the "Info is Power" series is its holistic approach to health and wellness. Instead of relying on a one-size-fits-all solution, Irene A. York delves into the intricacies of each condition and tailors her advice to offer a unique battle strategy. By incorporating a combination of natural remedies, cutting-edge techniques, and therapeutic modalities, the series provides readers with a comprehensive toolkit to address the multifaceted aspects of their health challenges.

"Cookin' with Cannabis," for example, dives into the world of culinary delights infused with cannabis, offering readers an opportunity to explore the healing potential of this remarkable plant. "Attack Arthritis" and "Combat Chronic Pain" focus on managing these debilitating conditions, bringing relief through a blend of cannabis use and therapeutic practices. In "Battle Beastly Bowels," you'll discover strategies to take control of digestive issues that often disrupt daily life. "Defeat Depression Drama" explores innovative techniques to conquer the mental health challenges that weigh heavily on so many individuals. "Strategic Sleep Solutions" offers guidance on overcoming sleep disturbances, a common but underestimated health problem.

One of the standout elements of the "Info is Power" series is the integration of cannabis as a powerful tool for health and wellness. Cannabis, a versatile plant with numerous therapeutic properties, has been gaining recognition for its potential to alleviate various health conditions. Irene A. York's books provide invaluable insights into the responsible and informed use of cannabis, including its various strains, methods of consumption, and potential benefits. By demystifying the world of cannabis, the series allows readers to harness its healing power in a safe and effective manner.

In addition to cannabis, the "Info is Power" series incorporates the transformative techniques of neuro-linguistic programming (NLP) and hypnosis. These psychological tools are explored in detail, offering readers the ability to reframe their thoughts and beliefs, ultimately leading to positive behavioral changes. By combining these therapeutic methods with cannabis, the series offers a comprehensive approach to health and wellness.

When you embark on your journey with the "Info is Power" series, you're not just reading a book; you're entering a realm of empowerment and self-discovery. Irene's friendly tone and deep empathy for those facing health challenges make her books approachable and relatable. Her experience shines through each page, giving you the confidence to tackle your health hurdles head-on.

To embark on your own journey to reclaim your health and well-being, you can find and purchase your favorite titles from the "Info is Power" series on Amazon by following this link: https://amzn.to/3rRpAOD.

In conclusion, the "Info is Power" series by Green Irene, aka Irene A. York, is an extraordinary collection of books and guides that empowers individuals facing chronic aches and pains, illness, or disease. With a focus on cannabis, NLP, and hypnosis, each title offers a tailored battle strategy to help you take control of your health and improve your quality of life. Don't miss the opportunity to transform your health journey; dive into these insightful resources and discover the power of information in the pursuit of well-being.

# Titles to review include:

- Attack Arthritis
- Battle Beastly Bowels
- Combat Chronic Pain
- Cookin' with Cannabis for a Medicated Day
- CBGTV's Bud Break – Compilation of Strain Reviews
- Cannabis Consumption Companion Journals
- Battle Strategy Journals
- Defeat Depression Drama
- Elevate Endogenous Health & Wellness
- Fight Fibro Green & Clean
- Tincture Time
- Strategic Sleep Solutions

**AND MORE!**

.

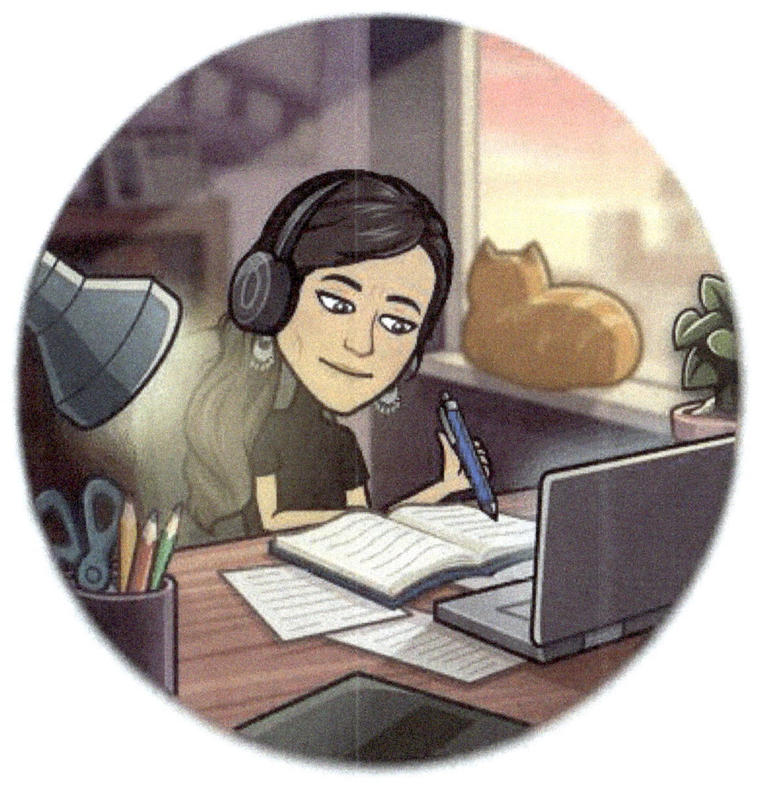

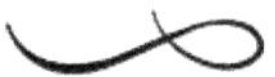

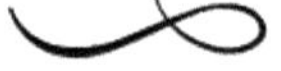